The Ultimate
Egg Bites

Delicious Egg Bites You Can Make At Home With An Egg Bites Maker

Marilyn Haugen

With

Jennifer Williams

Emjay Media Productions

ISBN: 978-0-9982470-3-8

PUBLISHERS NOTES

Disclaimer

This publication is intended to provide helpful and informative material. It is not intended to diagnose, treat, cure, or prevent any health problem or condition, nor is intended to replace the advice of a physician. No action should be taken solely on the contents of this book. Always consult your physician or qualified health-care professional on any matters regarding your health and before adopting any suggestions in this book or drawing inferences from it.

The author and publisher specifically disclaim all responsibility for any liability, loss or risk, personal or otherwise, which is incurred as a consequence, directly or indirectly, from the use or application of any contents of this book.

Any and all product names referenced within this book are the trademarks of their respective owners. None of these owners have sponsored, authorized, endorsed, or approved this book. The author is not associated with * Hamilton Beach Brands, Inc.® or Starbucks® is a registered trademark of Starbucks Corporation. Use of the Hamilton Beach trademark or the Starbucks trademark does not imply any affiliation with or endorsement by their respective corporations.

Always read all information provided by the manufacturers' product labels before using their products. The author and publisher are not responsible for claims made by manufacturers.

Paperback Edition   Manufactured in the United States of America

TABLE OF CONTENTS

ACKNOWLEDGMENTS

To all the wonderful women in my life; my daughter, mother, grandmothers, relatives and friends. You have taught me, supported me and loved me throughout my journeys. You are all amazing women.

Introduction

When sous vide egg bites were first introduced on to the breakfast scene by Starbucks several years ago, I don't know if anyone imagined how popular these little bites would become. Well now we can make them faster, with more options, and at much less expense than the original.

There are numerous "sous vide" egg bite copycat recipes all over the internet. Many use an Instant Pot or make them in muffin tins in the oven. However, I have found nothing quite as simple, delicious and foolproof as using an egg bites maker to make egg bites.

My brand of choice is the Hamilton Beach Egg Bites Maker. The recipes are designed to go with that maker, but other egg bites makers will work just as well.

With these delicious recipes and an egg bites maker, your morning meal couldn't be quicker or more delicious. The recipes are easy to make, ready in 5 minutes and clean-up is a breeze.

Breakfast is often the hardest meal to fit into your schedule or to figure out what to make. This handy little appliance makes it so easy. Plus, egg bites can be made ahead of time, tightly sealed and refrigerated.

In addition to egg bites, you can make poached eggs, and with some models also can make boiled eggs. We've included recipes for your favorite poached egg dishes, such as Eggs Benedict.

A great breakfast gives your body essential fuel and nutrients to power you through the day. Top this off with your favorite juice, a glass of milk, and an amazing cup of coffee and you should be ready to kick off your day.

All recipes use the Egg Bites Maker from TM & Copywrite Hamilton Beach Brands, Inc. to make these delicious egg dishes in under 10 minutes. Any other similar egg bites makers can be used with modifications for the specific appliance following the manufacturer's instructions.

Getting Started

The recipes in this book have been designed to work with an Egg Bites maker. You will find some of the directions very similar between recipes. That is because it just takes a few simple steps to get your egg bite or poached egg ready to eat. Also, I personally do not like reading a recipe that continually refers me back to the appliance manufacturer's instructions of some other random place – I want it all in one spot – hopefully you will too.

Our Go-To Small Appliance: Hamilton Beach Egg Bites Maker

Using the Hamilton Beach Egg Bites Maker is a breeze. No preheating is needed. Just get your ingredients ready and you're good to go. This small appliance steams your egg bites, locking in flavor and moisture. It's efficient and saves you time in the kitchen.

The recipes in this book will also work very well with other egg bites makers. About the only things we have found different are the heating and filling instructions – although they are all very similar.

Supplies List

- ✓ Hamilton Beach Egg Bites Maker (or other Egg Bites Makers)
- ✓ Small single-serve blender or whisk and bowl
- ✓ Silicone or wooden spatula
- ✓ Measuring cups and spoons

Initial Setup

1. **Set the maker up**: Put it on a stable surface, near an outlet, but not close to anything that the escaping steam could harm.
2. **Do not preheat:** Only plug in the maker after the egg bites are in the tray.
3. **Water first:** Add the required amount of water for cooking.

Basic Steps

1. **Blend or Whisk:** Use a blender or whisk to mix your eggs and add-ins.
2. **Fill the tray:** Pour your mixture into the egg tray up to the fill line.
3. **Start cooking:** Close the lid and plug the egg bites maker in.
4. **Times up:** The egg bites are ready when the green light shuts off. For egg bites, this takes about 5 minutes.
5. **Let rest:** Let the egg bites or poached eggs stand about 2 to 3 minutes before removing them from the molds. This step gives them time to firm up a little.

Ingredients

Eggs: Large eggs or liquid egg whites are used.

Meat: When adding meat, the most common ingredients are diced ham, bacon or sausage. Occasionally, we use Canadian bacon, smoked salmon, prosciutto or other specialty meats, particularly in our Eggs Benedict and variations.

Dairy: The most common foundational dairy we use is cottage cheese, cream cheese, milk or cream. These can be substituted with your favorite non-dairy version of these ingredients. Some, but not all, of the recipes call for shredded cheese. Here too, you can use your favorite non-dairy version. However, there are also a number of recipes that do not call for additional cheese.

Vegetables: The vegetables used in the recipes are often interchangeable with ones that you prefer. In many cases, the recipe is a great way to use up leftover cooked vegetables. You can also use defrosted frozen vegetables in place of fresh.

Safety Pointers

- ✓ Follow the manufacturer's instructions on how to handle your machine. They know best what works and what does not.
- ✓ Be careful when handling the machine or trays when they are hot. Keep your hands away from the egg cooker while it is cooking since steam can escape. Use oven mitts when opening the lid.
- ✓ If children are involved, adult supervision is a must.

Cleanup Made Easy

1. **Power Off:** Turn off the machine when cooking is done.
2. **Cooling Down Time:** Wait for the machine to cool before you clean.
3. **Easy Clean:** The tray is dishwasher safe. The egg bites tray is also easy to clean with soap and water. Wipe the maker with a damp cloth.

You've got the basics down. Now explore the recipes and get cooking!

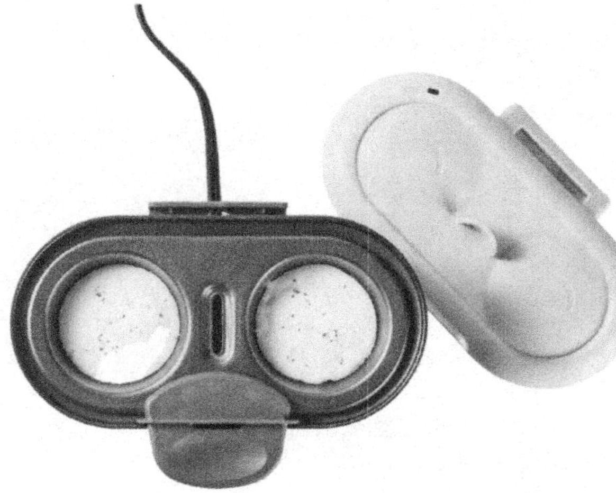

Not only is an egg bites maker good for making egg bites, but many of them can also poach eggs, boil eggs, or make omelets.

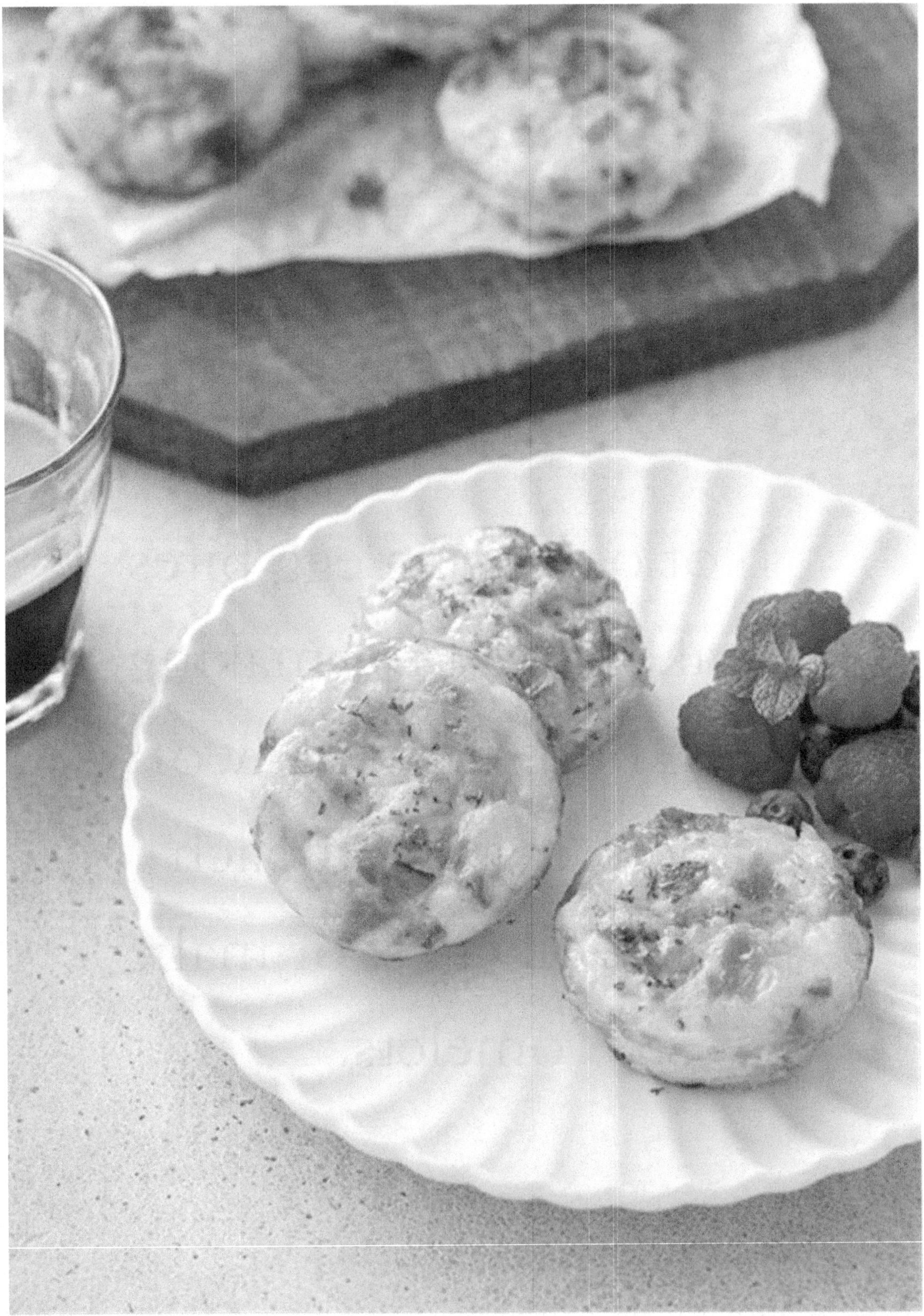

Classic Bites

Prep Tips

For small portions of chopped or diced onions, peppers, tomatoes, mushrooms, olives, bacon, etc., stop by the takeout or salad buffet section of your grocery store. You will find an array of fresh fixings you can put in your egg bites. Plus, you can purchase only what you need.

Bacon & Cheddar Bites

Savor the timeless pairing of crispy bacon and rich cheddar with our Bacon & Cheddar Bites recipe, tailored for the Sous Vide Style Electric Egg Bite Maker & Poacher. These tasty and effortless egg bites are ready in just 10 minutes. A must-have for a quick on-the-go breakfast.

Serving Size: 2 egg bites | Prep Time: 3 Minutes | Cook Time: 7 Minutes

---

Ingredients:

1	large egg
2 tbsp.	cottage cheese
3 tbsp.	shredded cheddar cheese
Pinch	kosher salt and freshly ground black pepper
2 tbsp.	cooked and crumbled bacon

Instructions:

1. Using a personal blender, combine the egg, cottage cheese and 2 tbsp. cheddar cheese, salt and black pepper.
2. Sprinkle half the remaining cheddar and half of the bacon into each mold.
3. Pour the egg mixture evenly into the egg bite molds up to the "Max" fill line.
4. Fill the egg bite maker with water according to the manufacturer's directions.
5. Place the mold in the cooker and close the lid. Plug in the egg cooker.
6. After about 7 minutes, or when the green light turns off, carefully remove the egg tray from the cooker.
7. Let stand a few minutes. Then invert the egg bites on to a serving plate.

Tip

- 2 slices of bacon are equal to 2 tbsp. of cooked and crumbled bacon.

Famous Bacon and Gruyère Bites

This famous combination of bacon and gruyere made into a grab and go egg bite was the one from Starbucks that inspired it all. It's simple, oh so tasty and can be made at home faster and less expensively.

Serving Size: 2 egg bites | Preparation Time: 3 minutes | Cooking Time: 7 minutes

Ingredients:

1	large egg
3 tbsp.	cottage cheese
2 tbsp.	shredded Gruyère
Pinch	kosher salt and freshly ground black pepper
1 tbsp.	diced bacon

Instructions

1. Using a personal blender, combine the egg, cottage cheese, half of the Gruyère, salt and pepper.
2. Sprinkle half the remaining Gruyère and half of the bacon into each mold.
3. Pour the egg mixture evenly into the egg bite molds up to the "Max" fill line.
4. Fill the egg bite maker with water according to the manufacturer's directions.
5. Place the mold in the cooker and close the lid. Plug in the egg cooker.
6. After about 7 minutes, or when the green light turns off, carefully remove the egg tray from the cooker.
7. Let stand a few minutes. Then invert the egg bites on to a serving plate.

Tip:

- Substitute Gruyère with Monterey Jack if you prefer. Or use half of each.

Tex-Mex Fiesta Bites

Savor the vibrant flavors of this delightful recipe that brings together zesty Tex-Mex ingredients in one delicious dish. Create a Tex-Mex fiesta in your kitchen with these easy-to-make bites.

Serving Size: 2 egg bites | Preparation Time: 3 minutes | Cooking Time: 7 minutes

Ingredients:

1	large egg
2 tbsp.	sour cream
2 tbsp.	shredded pepper jack cheese
1 tbsp.	crumbled cooked chorizo
Pinch	kosher salt and freshly ground black pepper
1 tbsp.	chopped tomatoes (about 2 cherry tomatoes)
1-1/2 tsp.	chopped fresh cilantro

Instructions:

1. Using a personal blender, combine the egg, sour cream, pepper jack cheese, chorizo, salt and pepper.
2. Divide the tomatoes and the cilantro into each egg bite mold.
3. Pour the egg mixture evenly into the egg bite molds up to the "Max" fill line.
4. Fill the egg bite maker with water according to the manufacturer's directions.
5. Place the mold in the cooker and close the lid. Plug in the egg cooker.
6. After about 7 minutes, or when the green light turns off, carefully remove the egg tray from the cooker.
7. Let stand a few minutes. Then invert the egg bites on to a serving plate.

Tips:

- Use any variety of spicy sausage you have on hand in place of the chorizo.

BREAKFAST TACO

Double up on your favorite foods with this egg bite breakfast taco. All you need are the Tex Mex Fiesta bites, a softened taco sized tortilla, some salsa and optional black beans for an extra protein kick.

Serving Size: 2 egg bites | Preparation Time: 3 minutes | Cooking Time: 7 minutes

Ingredients:

2	Tex-Mex Fiesta Bites
1	taco size flour tortilla
2 tbsp.	warmed black beans
2 tbsp.	salsa
1 -2 tbsp.	shredded Mexican cheese blend
	Sour cream (optional)

Instructions:

1. Prepare the Tex-Mex Fiesta bites as directed above.
2. Warm the tortilla in a large skillet or wrapped in a damp paper towel in the microwave.
3. Lay the tortilla on a flat surface. Spoon black beans down the middle of the tortilla.
4. Add the 2 egg bites on top of the beans.
5. Spoon salsa on top of the egg bites. Sprinkle with cheese blend.
6. Tightly roll up the taco.
7. Serve with a dollop of sour cream, if using.

Tips:

- Use 2 street size taco tortillas in place of the regular size and divide the ingredients between each.
- If you would like more room for your fillers, use an enchilada size tortilla.

Lox & Cream Cheese Pleaser

Try this delicious recipe that pairs cream cheese with savory lox. Almost like your favorite deli but without the bagel.

Serving Size: 2 egg bites | Preparation Time: 3 minutes | Cooking Time: 7 minutes

Ingredients:

3 tbsp.	liquid egg whites
2 tbsp.	cottage cheese
1 tbsp.	cream cheese, softened
Pinch	kosher salt and freshly ground black pepper
1 oz.	lox, cut into small chunks
2 tsp.	chopped chives
	Capers (optional)

Instructions:

1. Using a personal blender, combine the egg whites, cottage cheese, cream cheese, salt and pepper.
1. Divide the lox and chives into each egg bite mold.
2. Pour the egg mixture evenly on top of the lox and chives into the egg bite molds up to the "Max" fill line.
3. Fill the egg bite maker with water according to the manufacturer's directions.
4. Place the mold in the cooker and close the lid. Plug in the egg cooker.
5. After about 7 minutes, or when the green light turns off, carefully remove the egg tray from the cooker.
6. Let stand a few minutes. Then invert the egg bites on to a serving plate.
7. Garnish with capers, if using.

Tips:

- 1 oz. of lox is about 2 to 3 tbsp. of crumbled lox depending on the density of the lox. 3 tbsp. is the ideal amount for this recipe, so adjust the ounces accordingly.
- For simplicity, use chive and cream cheese spread in place of the cream cheese and chives.
- Add the egg bites to a bagel with cream cheese shmeer.

HAM & GOUDA BLISS

Ham and gouda make a delicious pairing of salty, savory, smoky and creamy all rolled up into two delicious egg bites. They are so tasty you may want to make a more for later.

Serving Size: 2 egg bites | Preparation Time: 3 minutes | Cooking Time: 7 minutes

---

Ingredients:

1	large egg
2 tbsp.	cottage cheese
3 tbsp.	diced cooked ham
2 tbsp.	shredded Gouda cheese
Pinch	kosher salt and freshly ground black pepper

Instructions:

1. Using a personal blender, combine the egg, cottage cheese, half of the diced ham, half of the Gouda, salt and pepper.
2. Divide the remaining ham and cheese into each egg bite mold.
3. Pour the egg mixture evenly into the egg bite molds up to the "Max" fill line.
4. Fill the egg bite maker with water according to the manufacturer's directions.
5. Place the mold in the cooker and close the lid. Plug in the egg cooker.
6. After about 7 minutes, or when the green light turns off, carefully remove the egg tray from the cooker.
7. Let stand a few minutes. Then invert the egg bites on to a serving plate.

Tip:

- Add some smoky flavor by using smoked Gouda cheese.

Buffalo Chicken Egg Bites

Lover's off buffalo chicken this is your breakfast home run. Shredded chicken, cheese, and buffalo sauce are all equally delicious in egg bites. You may even want to make these for game day snacks.

Serving Size: 2 egg bites | Preparation Time: 5 minutes | Cooking Time: 7 minutes

---

Ingredients:

1	large egg
2 tbsp.	cottage cheese
2 tbsp.	shredded rotisserie chicken
2 tsp.	buffalo sauce
Pinch	kosher salt
2 tbsp.	shredded Mexican cheese blend
2 tsp.	chopped green onions

Instructions:

1. Using a personal blender, combine the egg, cottage cheese, chicken, buffalo sauce, salt, half of the cheese blend and half of the green onions.
2. Divide the remaining cheese blend and onions into each egg bite mold.
3. Pour the egg mixture evenly into the egg bite molds up to the "Max" fill line.
4. Fill the egg bite maker with water according to the manufacturer's directions.
5. Place the mold in the cooker and close the lid. Plug in the egg cooker.
6. After about 7 minutes, or when the green light turns off, carefully remove the egg tray from the cooker.
7. Let stand a few minutes. Then invert the egg bites on to a serving plate.

Tips:

- Instead of leftover rotisserie chicken, use a packet or can of shredded chicken.

Broccoli & Ham Quiche Bites

Simple, yet perfect quiche in an egg bite. A delicious combination of broccoli, ham, and Swiss cheese. A great option for using leftover ham and steamed broccoli.

Serving Size: 2 egg bites | Preparation Time: 5 minutes | Cooking Time: 7 minutes

Ingredients:

1	large egg
1 tbsp.	cottage cheese
2 tbsp.	diced cooked ham
2 tbsp.	chopped frozen broccoli, thawed
2 tbsp.	shredded cheese
	Parsley flakes
	Kosher salt and freshly ground black pepper

Instructions:

1. Using a personal blender, combine the egg, cottage cheese, half of the ham, half of the broccoli, half of the Swiss cheese, parsley flakes, salt and pepper.
2. Divide the remaining ham, broccoli and Swiss cheese into each egg bite mold.
3. Pour the egg mixture evenly into the egg bite molds up to the "Max" fill line.
4. Fill the egg bite maker with water according to the manufacturer's directions.
5. Place the mold in the cooker and close the lid. Plug in the egg cooker.
6. After about 7 minutes, or when the green light turns off, carefully remove the egg tray from the cooker.
7. Let stand a few minutes. Then invert the egg bites on to a serving plate.

Tips:

- Use leftover cooked broccoli when possible.
- Defrost a frozen package of chopped steamed broccoli and divide it into ice cube trays and refrigerate or refreeze for perfectly sized portions.

BACON, SPINACH & PEPPER JACK BITES

Add a little bite to your morning eggs with pepper Jack cheese. Paired with steamed spinach and chopped bacon, it is a great pick-me-up in the morning.

Serving Size: 2 egg bites | Preparation Time: 3 minutes | Cooking Time: 7 minutes

Ingredients:

1	large egg
2 tbsp.	cottage cheese
1 tbsp.	chopped cooked spinach
2 tbsp.	cooked and crumbled bacon
2 tbsp.	shredded Pepper Jack cheese
Pinch	kosher salt

Instructions:

1. Using a personal blender, combine the egg, cottage cheese, the spinach, half of the bacon, half of the half of the pepper Jack cheese and salt.
2. Divide the remaining bacon and cheese into each egg bite mold.
3. Pour the egg mixture evenly into the egg bite molds up to the "Max" fill line.
4. Fill the egg bite maker with water according to the manufacturer's directions.
5. Place the mold in the cooker and close the lid. Plug in the egg cooker.
6. After about 7 minutes, or when the green light turns off, carefully remove the egg tray from the cooker.
7. Let stand a few minutes. Then invert the egg bites on to a serving plate.

Tips:

- 2 sliced cooked bacon equals about 2 tbsp. cooked and crumbled bacon.
- Use real bacon bits for simplicity.

EGGS BENEDICT BITES

When you want to treat yourself in the morning, eggs benedict is the go-to dish of many. But when you don't have time to spare, these Eggs Benedict bites come very close to perfection.

Serving Size: 2 egg bites | Preparation Time: 3 minutes | Cooking Time: 7 minutes

---

Ingredients:

1	large egg
2 tbsp.	cottage cheese
1 tbsp.	onion flakes
Pinch	kosher salt
Pinch	paprika
Pinch	ground nutmeg
2 tbsp.	chopped Canadian bacon
2 tbsp.	shredded Gruyere cheese

Instructions:

1. Using a personal blender, combine the egg, cottage cheese, onion flakes, salt, paprika, nutmeg, half of the bacon and half of the Gruyere.
2. Divide the remaining bacon and Gruyere into each egg bite mold.
3. Pour the egg mixture evenly into the egg bite molds up to the "Max" fill line.
4. Fill the egg bite maker with water according to the manufacturer's directions.
5. Place the mold in the cooker and close the lid. Plug in the egg cooker.
6. After about 7 minutes, or when the green light turns off, carefully remove the egg tray from the cooker.
7. Let stand a few minutes. Then invert the egg bites on to a serving plate.

Tips:

- Feel free to use shredded white cheddar in place of the Gruyere.
- Another option is to use crumbled bacon instead of Canadian bacon.
- Add the egg bites to a toasted English muffin for a nice variation. You can even make them into a breakfast sandwich using the whole English muffin.

SMOKED SALMON & DILL BITES

Smoked salmon and dill are a classic combination that is hard to resist. Now you can enjoy that exquisite taste in an egg bite.

Serving Size: 2 egg bites | Preparation Time: 5 minutes | Cooking Time: 7 minutes

Ingredients:

1	large egg
2 tbsp.	cottage cheese
1 oz	smoked salmon, chopped (about 2 tbsp.)
2 tbsp.	capers, drained
Pinch	Freshly ground black pepper
1/2 tbsp.	chopped fresh dill

Instructions:

1. Using a personal blender, combine the egg, cottage cheese, smoked salmon, half of the capers and the pepper.
2. Divide remaining capers and the dill into the bottom of the egg bites mold.
3. Pour the egg mixture evenly into the molds up to the "Max" fill line.
4. Fill the egg bite maker with water according to the manufacturer's directions.
5. Place the mold in the cooker and close the lid. Plug in the egg cooker.
6. After about 7 minutes, or when the green light turns off, carefully remove the egg tray from the cooker.
7. Let stand a few minutes. Then invert the egg bites on to a serving plate.

Tips:

- Substitute 3 egg whites for the 1 large egg.
- Sprinkle with Everything But the Bagel Seasoning before serving.

Sausage & Mushroom Egg Bites

Mushrooms make a tasty egg bite into an umami powerhouse. The taste, texture and nutrient values make a great combination to start the day.

Serving Size: 2 egg bites | Preparation Time: 5 minutes | Cooking Time: 7 minutes

Ingredients:

1	large egg
2 tbsp.	cottage cheese
2 tbsp.	cooked and crumbled breakfast sausage
2 tbsp.	sliced mushrooms
Pinch	Kosher salt and freshly ground black pepper
1/2 tbsp.	chopped fresh parsley

Instructions:

1. Using a personal blender, combine the egg and cottage cheese. Add the breakfast sausage, mushrooms, salt and pepper and pulse the blender a couple of times until just combined.
2. Sprinkle the fresh parsley into the bottom of the egg bite molds.
3. Pour the egg mixture evenly into the molds up to the "Max" fill line.
4. Fill the egg bite maker with water according to the manufacturer's directions.
5. Place the mold in the cooker and close the lid. Plug in the egg cooker.
6. After about 7 minutes, or when the green light turns off, carefully remove the egg tray from the cooker.
7. Let stand a few minutes. Then invert the egg bites on to a serving plate.

Tips:

- 1/4 of a cooked breakfast sausage patty equals about 2 tbsp. of crumbled sausage.
- Do not over blend the sausage and mushrooms with the egg mixture. You want the pieces to be coarse and visible.

Sausage & Bell Pepper Fiesta

Spice up your morning routine with our Sausage & Bell Pepper Fiesta recipe. These zesty egg bites are a real fiesta for your taste buds.

Serving Size: 2 egg bites | Preparation Time: 5 minutes | Cooking Time: 7 minutes

---

Ingredients:

1	large egg
2 tbsp.	cottage cheese
2 tbsp.	cooked sausage crumbles
2 tbsp.	diced sweet peppers (assorted colors)
Pinch	Kosher salt and freshly ground black pepper
1 tbsp.	shredded cheddar cheese

Instructions:

1. Using a personal blender, combine the egg and cottage cheese. Add the breakfast sausage, sweet peppers, salt and pepper and pulse the blender a couple of times.
2. Sprinkle the cheddar cheese evenly divided into the bottom of the egg bite molds.
3. Pour the egg mixture evenly into the molds up to the "Max" fill line.
4. Fill the egg bite maker with water according to the manufacturer's directions.
5. Place the mold in the cooker and close the lid. Plug in the egg cooker.
6. After about 7 minutes, or when the green light turns off, carefully remove the egg tray from the cooker.
7. Let stand a few minutes. Then invert the egg bites on to a serving plate.

Tip:

- Make sure not to over blend the sausage and peppers. The added texture adds to the tastiness of these egg bites.

Canadian Bacon & Swiss

Ham and Swiss are a classic combination, so here we paired Swiss cheese with Canadian bacon for equally appealing results.

Serving Size: 2 egg bites | Preparation Time: 3 minutes | Cooking Time: 7 minutes

Ingredients:

1	large egg
2 tbsp.	cottage cheese
1 tsp.	Dijon mustard
Pinch	Kosher salt and freshly ground black pepper
2 tbsp.	diced Canadian bacon, about 2 round slices
2 tbsp.	shredded Swiss cheese

Instructions:

1. Using a personal blender, combine the egg, cottage cheese, Dijon mustard, salt and pepper. Add half of the Canadian bacon and the Swiss cheese and pulse the blender a couple of times.
2. Sprinkle the remaining Canadian bacon and Swiss cheese evenly divided into the bottom of the egg bite molds.
3. Pour the egg mixture evenly into the molds up to the "Max" fill line.
4. Fill the egg bite maker with water according to the manufacturer's directions.
5. Place the mold in the cooker and close the lid. Plug in the egg cooker.
6. After about 7 minutes, or when the green light turns off, carefully remove the egg tray from the cooker.
7. Let stand a few minutes. Then invert the egg bites on to a serving plate.

Tip:

- Use regular chopped ham in place of the Canadian bacon, if desired.

Black Forest Ham & Asparagus

Black Forest ham is very moist and has a deep rich flavor from the wood used in smoking. This all comes together with asparagus and Gouda cheese in little egg bites.

Serving Size: 2 egg bites | Preparation Time: 3 minutes | Cooking Time: 7 minutes

---

Ingredients:

1	large egg
2 tbsp.	diced Black Forest ham
2 tbsp.	steamed asparagus tips
2 tbsp.	Gouda cheese, shredded
1 tbsp.	heavy cream
	Kosher salt and freshly ground black pepper

Instructions:

1. Using a personal blender, combine the egg, cottage cheese, Dijon mustard, salt and pepper. Add half of the Canadian bacon and the Swiss cheese and pulse the blender a couple of times.
2. Sprinkle the remaining Canadian bacon and Swiss cheese evenly divided into the bottom of the egg bite molds.
3. Pour the egg mixture evenly into the molds up to the "Max" fill line.
4. Fill the egg bite maker with water according to the manufacturer's directions.
5. Place the mold in the cooker and close the lid. Plug in the egg cooker.
6. After about 7 minutes, or when the green light turns off, carefully remove the egg tray from the cooker.
7. Let stand a few minutes. Then invert the egg bites on to a serving plate.

Tips:

- Use frozen steamed asparagus tips and defrost them before using. Pull out as much as you need from the package and return the remainder to the freezer.
- You can also find cooked asparagus in jars or cans. Leftovers can be covered and refrigerated for up to 1 week.

SWEET POTATO & TURKEY BACON

A year-round egg bite that reminds you of the classic flavors of Thanksgiving all in two tasty bites.

Serving Size: 2 egg bites | Preparation Time: 3 minutes | Cooking Time: 7 minutes

Ingredients:

1	large egg
1 tbsp.	cottage cheese
2 tbsp.	roasted sweet potatoes, diced
Pinch	kosher salt and freshly ground black pepper
2 tbsp.	chopped cooked turkey bacon
2 tbsp.	shredded sharp cheddar cheese

Instructions:

1. Using a personal blender, combine the egg, cottage cheese, sweet potatoes, salt and pepper. Add half of the turkey bacon and the cheddar cheese and pulse the blender a couple of times.
2. Sprinkle the remaining Canadian bacon and Swiss cheese evenly divided into the bottom of the egg bite molds.
3. Pour the egg mixture evenly into the molds up to the "Max" fill line.
4. Fill the egg bite maker with water according to the manufacturer's directions.
5. Place the mold in the cooker and close the lid. Plug in the egg cooker.
6. After about 7 minutes, or when the green light turns off, carefully remove the egg tray from the cooker.
7. Let stand a few minutes. Then invert the egg bites on to a serving plate.

Tip:

- Set aside some leftover roasted sweet potatoes from another meal to be used in this recipe.
- You can also use 2 tbsp. of leftover shredded cooked turkey if you prefer. Put all the turkey in the blender and do not set any aside to put directly into the molds.

Festive Turkey & Cranberry

These egg bites feature the classic combination of tender turkey and tart cranberries. Who says you have to wait until the holidays to enjoy this combination.

Serving Size: 2 egg bites | Preparation Time: 3 minutes | Cooking Time: 7 minutes

---

Ingredients:

1	large egg
2 tbsp.	chopped cooked turkey breast
2 tbsp.	dried cranberries
2 tbsp.	shredded Gouda cheese
1 tbsp.	cottage cheese
Pinch	kosher salt and freshly ground black pepper

Instructions:

1. Using a personal blender, combine the egg, chopped cooked turkey breast, dried cranberries, shredded Gouda, cottage cheese, salt and pepper.
2. Pour the mixture evenly into the egg bite molds, filling them up to the "Max" fill line.
3. Fill the egg bite maker with water according to the manufacturer's directions.
4. Place the mold in the egg bite maker and securely close the lid. Plug in the egg cooker.
5. After approximately 7 minutes, or when the green light turns off, carefully remove the egg tray from the cooker.
6. Allow the egg bites to stand for a few minutes to cool slightly.
7. Gently invert the egg bites onto a serving plate.

Tip:

- Serve egg bites on a cornbread muffin or with leftover stuffing.

RAGIN' CAJUN BITES

Take a trip to Cajun country with this morning dose of andouille sausage, jalapenos, and eggs whites to start your day with a wallop.

Serving Size: 2 egg bites | Preparation Time: 3 minutes | Cooking Time: 7 minutes

---

Ingredients:

3 tbsp.	liquid egg whites
2 tbsp.	cottage cheese
1/8 tsp.	garlic powder
Pinch	kosher salt and freshly ground black pepper
2 tbsp.	crumbled cooked andouille sausage
2 tbsp.	shredded cheddar cheese
1 tsp.	diced Jalapenos, plus more for garnish

Instructions:

1. Using a personal blender, combine the egg whites, cottage cheese, garlic powder, salt and pepper. Add half of the andouille sausage and half of the cheddar cheese and pulse the blender a couple of times.
2. Sprinkle the remaining sausage and cheese evenly divided into the bottom of the egg bite molds.
3. Pour the egg mixture evenly into the molds up to the "Max" fill line.
4. Fill the egg bite maker with water according to the manufacturer's directions.
5. Place the mold in the egg bite maker and securely close the lid. Plug in the egg cooker.
6. After approximately 7 minutes, or when the green light turns off, carefully remove the egg tray from the cooker.
7. Allow the egg bites to stand for a few minutes to cool slightly.
8. Gently invert the egg bites onto a serving plate.
9. Garnish with diced Jalapenos or a thin slice of Jalapeno on each egg bite.

Tip:

- For a spicier taste, add a Pinch of hot sauce, such as Frank's Red Hot in step 1. You can also serve the hot sauce alongside so everyone can add their own.

MONTE CRISTO BITES

A favorite sandwich of ham, turkey swiss and seasonings all packed into egg bites. Get ready for dipping in a little strawberry jam and powdered sugar.

Serving Size: 2 egg bites | Preparation Time: 3 minutes | Cooking Time: 7 minutes

Ingredients:

1	large egg
1 tbsp.	sour cream
1 tsp.	Dijon mustard
Pinch	ground nutmeg
Pinch	Kosher salt and freshly ground black pepper
2 tbsp.	chopped ham
2 tbsp.	chopped turkey
2 tbsp.	shredded Swiss cheese
	Powdered sugar (optional)
	Strawberry jam (optional)

Instructions:

1. Using a personal blender, combine the egg, sour cream, mustard, nutmeg, salt and pepper. Add half of the ham, turkey and Swiss and pulse the blender a couple of times.
2. Sprinkle the remaining ham, turkey and Swiss evenly divided into the bottom of the egg bite molds.
3. Pour the egg mixture evenly into the molds up to the "Max" fill line.
4. Fill the egg bite maker with water according to the manufacturer's directions.
5. Place the mold in the egg bite maker and securely close the lid. Plug in the egg cooker.
6. After approximately 7 minutes, or when the green light turns off, carefully remove the egg tray from the cooker.
7. Allow the egg bites to stand for a few minutes to cool slightly.
8. Gently invert the egg bites onto a serving plate.
9. Serve egg bites with powdered sugar and strawberry jam, is using.

Tip:

- After you put half of the chopped ham and turkey into the blender, make sure the remainder is finely chopped before adding them to the molds.

Leek, Bacon & Cheese Mini Frittatas

No need for a large frittata, when you can get the same flavors for breakfast with these tasty little egg bites.

Serving Size: 2 egg bites | Preparation Time: 3 minutes | Cooking Time: 7 minutes

---

Ingredients:

1	large egg
2 tbsp.	cottage cheese
1/2 tsp.	finely chopped fresh dill
Pinch	paprika
	Kosher salt and freshly ground black pepper
2 tbsp.	chopped cooked bacon
2 tbsp.	shredded white cheddar cheese
1 tbsp.	chopped leeks, white part only

Instructions:

1. Using a personal blender, combine the egg, cottage cheese, dill, salt and pepper. Add half the bacon, half the cheese and all the leeks to the blender. Pulse a couple of times just to combine.
2. Sprinkle the remaining bacon and cheese evenly divided into the egg molds.
3. Pour the egg mixture evenly into the molds up to the "Max" fill line.
4. Fill the egg bite maker with water according to the manufacturer's directions.
5. Place the mold in the egg bite maker and securely close the lid. Plug in the egg cooker.
6. After approximately 7 minutes, or when the green light turns off, carefully remove the egg tray from the cooker.
7. Allow the egg bites to stand for a few minutes to cool slightly.
8. Gently invert the egg bites onto a serving plate.

Tips:

- Substitute 3 tbsp. liquid eggs whites for the egg if you prefer.
- Use 1 tsp. dried leeks for the fresh leeks if desired.
- Use a pinch of dried dill in place of the fresh dill if desired.

Apple Gouda Chicken Bites

Gouda and real apple chunks give these chicken sausage bites a delicious, slightly sweet and slightly savory flavor. This delicious combination of flavors is easy to achieve using ready-made chicken sausage.

Serving Size: 2 egg bites | Preparation Time: 3 minutes | Cooking Time: 7 minutes

---

Ingredients:

3 tbsp	liquid egg bites
2 tbsp.	cottage cheese
Pinch	Kosher salt and freshly ground black pepper
Pinch	ground cinnamon (optional)
4 tbsp.	chopped cooked chicken sausage with apple and gouda

Instructions:

1. Using a personal blender, combine the egg whites, cottage cheese, salt, pepper and cinnamon, if using. Add 3 tbsp. of the sausage to the blender and pulse a couple of times just to combine.
2. Sprinkle the remaining sausage evenly divided into the egg molds.
3. Pour the egg mixture evenly into the molds up to the "Max" fill line.
4. Fill the egg bite maker with water according to the manufacturer's directions.
5. Place the mold in the egg bite maker and securely close the lid. Plug in the egg cooker.
6. After approximately 7 minutes, or when the green light turns off, carefully remove the egg tray from the cooker.
7. Allow the egg bites to stand for a few minutes to cool slightly.
8. Gently invert the egg bites onto a serving plate.

Tip:

- You can find Apple and Gouda Chicken sausage along with other types of refrigerated sausage. All brands I found were fully cooked. Check the label to be sure.

Apple Cheddar Bacon Egg Bites

Apple and cheddar are such a delightful combination at any time. So why not throw in a little bacon and make them into egg bites.

Serving Size: 2 egg bites | Preparation Time: 3 minutes | Cooking Time: 7 minutes

Ingredients:

1	large egg
2 tbsp.	cottage cheese
1 tsp.	French Toast Seasoning, plus more for garnish
Pinch	kosher salt
2 tbsp.	real bacon bits
2 tbsp.	shredded Monterey Jack cheese
2 tbsp.	chopped Granny Smith apple

Instructions:

1. Using a personal blender, combine the egg, cottage cheese, French toast seasoning and salt. Add the bacon bits, half of the cheese, and half of the apples to the blender. Pulse a couple of times just to combine.
2. Sprinkle the remaining cheese and apples evenly divided into the egg molds.
3. Pour the egg mixture evenly into the molds up to the "Max" fill line.
4. Fill the egg bite maker with water according to the manufacturer's directions.
5. Place the mold in the egg bite maker and securely close the lid. Plug in the egg cooker.
6. After approximately 7 minutes, or when the green light turns off, carefully remove the egg tray from the cooker.
7. Allow the egg bites to stand for a few minutes to cool slightly.
8. Gently invert the egg bites onto a serving plate.
9. Garnish with additional French Toast Seasoning, if desired

Tip:

- Substitute 3 tbsp. liquid eggs whites for the egg if you prefer.
- Make sure to buy **real** bacon bits. The other varieties are often made from flavored soybean meal and won't give you the desired result.

Aloha Chicken Bites

This recipe is so incredibly simple when you use a Aloha Chicken Sausage. The sausage is a delightful combination of seasoned chicken and pineapple. Don't be intimidate with this combination. The sausages are super easy to find and the marriage of flavors is irresistable.

Serving Size: 2 egg bites | Preparation Time: 3 minutes | Cooking Time: 7 minutes

---

Ingredients:

1	large egg
4 tbsp.	Aloha chicken sausage, crumbled
2 tbsp.	cream cheese, softened
Pinch	kosher salt and freshly ground black pepper

Instructions:

1. Using a personal blender, combine the egg, Aloha chicken sausage, cream cheese, salt and pepper.
2. Pour the egg mixture evenly into the molds up to the "Max" fill line.
3. Fill the egg bite maker with water according to the manufacturer's directions.
4. Place the mold in the cooker and close the lid. Plug in the egg cooker.
5. After about 7 minutes, or when the green light turns off, carefully remove the egg tray from the cooker.
6. Let stand a few minutes. Then invert the egg bites on to a serving plat

Tip:

Aloha chicken sausage is a specialty cooked sausage that can be found in the refrigerated sausage section in large grocery stores.

In place of the Aloha sausage, use 3 tbsp. chicken sausage, 1 tbsp. chopped canned pineapple and 1/8 tsp. minced ginger.

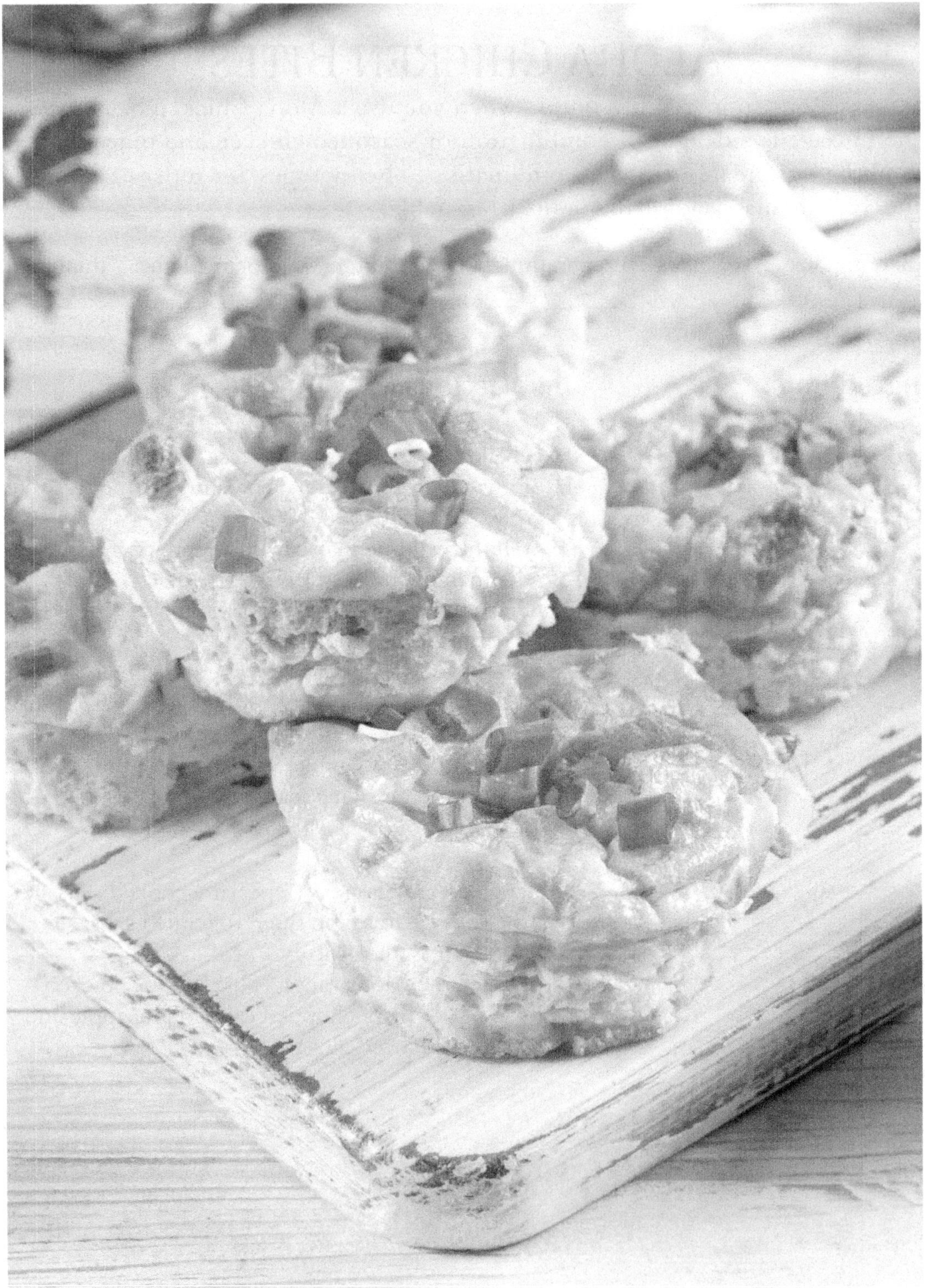

Vegetarian Bites

When using vegetables that have been frozen and defrosted, make sure to squezze out any excess moisture. Then, pat them dry with a paper towel.

Mediterranean Egg Bites

Capture the essence of Mediterranean flavors with a combination of feta cheese, black olives, bell peppers, and mint all blended into deliciously creamy egg bites.

Serving Size: 2 egg bites | Preparation Time: 5 minutes | Cooking Time: 7 minutes

---

Ingredients:

3 tbsp.	liquid egg whites
1 tbsp.	cream cheese, softened
1/2 tsp.	chopped fresh oregano
Pinch	kosher salt and freshly ground black pepper
2 tbsp.	diced mini peppers (any color)
2 tbsp.	crumbled feta cheese
2 tbsp.	sliced black or kalamata olives

Instructions:

1. Using a personal blender, combine the egg whites, cream cheese, oregano, salt and pepper. Add the mini peppers, half of the Feta, and half of the black olives to the blender. Pulse a couple of times just to combine.
2. Sprinkle the remaining feta and olives evenly divided into the egg molds.
3. Pour the egg mixture evenly into the molds up to the "Max" fill line.
4. Fill the egg bite maker with water according to the manufacturer's directions.
5. Place the mold in the egg bite maker and securely close the lid. Plug in the egg cooker.
6. After approximately 7 minutes, or when the green light turns off, carefully remove the egg tray from the cooker.
7. Allow the egg bites to stand for a few minutes to cool slightly.
8. Gently invert the egg bites onto a serving plate.

Tip:

Substitute 1 large egg for the egg whites if desired.

PESTO TOMATO & MOZZARELLA BITES

This classic combination of Italian flavors lightens up egg bites and adds a punch of flavor

Serving Size: 2 egg bites | Preparation Time: 3 minutes | Cooking Time: 7 minutes

Ingredients:

1	large egg
2 tbsp.	heavy cream
2 tsp.	pesto sauce
Pinch	kosher salt and freshly ground black pepper
2	cherry tomatoes, halved
2 tbsp.	fresh mozzarella pearls

Instructions:

1. Using a personal blender, combine the egg, heavy cream cheese, pesto sauce, salt and pepper. Add half of the cherry tomatoes and half of the fresh mozzarella to the blender. Pulse a couple of times just to combine.
2. Sprinkle the remaining cherry tomatoes and mozzarella pearls evenly divided into the egg molds.
3. Pour the egg mixture evenly into the molds up to the "Max" fill line.
4. Fill the egg bite maker with water according to the manufacturer's directions.
5. Place the mold in the egg bite maker and securely close the lid. Plug in the egg cooker.
6. After approximately 7 minutes, or when the green light turns off, carefully remove the egg tray from the cooker.
7. Allow the egg bites to stand for a few minutes .
8. Gently invert the egg bites onto a serving plate.

Tips:

- Use a couple of Ciliegine mozzarella balls or a chopped larger ball of fresh mozzarella in place of the pearls.
- Add more pesto sauce to taste.

Cheesy Spinach & Artichoke Bites

Almost like a favorite festive appetizer, but all bundled into tasty egg bites you can enjoy for breakfast or a snack.

Serving Size: 2 egg bites | Preparation Time: 5 minutes | Cooking Time: 7 minutes

Ingredients:

1	large egg
2 tbsp.	chopped cooked spinach (squeezed dry)
2 tbsp.	chopped canned artichoke hearts
2 tbsp.	shredded mozzarella cheese
1 tbsp.	cream cheese
Pinch	Kosher salt and freshly ground black pepper
1/2 tbsp.	grated fresh Parmesan cheese

Instructions:

1. Using a personal blender, combine the egg, spinach, artichoke hearts, mozzarella, creamed cheese, salt and pepper
2. Sprinkle the Parmesan cheese evenly divided into the egg molds.
3. Pour the egg mixture evenly into the molds up to the "Max" fill line.
4. Fill the egg bite maker with water according to the manufacturer's directions.
5. Place the mold in the egg bite maker and securely close the lid. Plug in the egg cooker.
6. After approximately 7 minutes, or when the green light turns off, carefully remove the egg tray from the cooker.
7. Allow the egg bites to stand for a few minutes to cool slightly.
8. Gently invert the egg bites onto a serving plate.

Tips:

- Cover and refrigerate leftover artichoke hearts for up to 5 days.
- Defrost a frozen package of chopped broccoli and divide it into ice cube trays and refrigerate or refreeze for perfectly sized portions.

Spinach Dip Bites

Everyone's favorite spinach dip all bundled into egg bites. Make two or make a dozen for party finger food. You won't be disappointed.

Serving Size: 2 egg bites | Preparation Time: 5 minutes | Cooking Time: 7 minutes

---

Ingredients:

1	large egg
2 tbsp.	chopped cooked spinach (squeezed dry)
2 tbsp.	sour cream
2 tbsp.	chopped water chestnuts
1 tbsp.	mayonnaise
1 tsp.	Knorr® Vegetable recipe mix
1/2 tsp.	dried green onion flakes

Instructions:

1. Using a personal blender, combine the egg, spinach, sour cream, water chestnuts, mayonnaise, the dried vegetable mix, and the green onion flakes.
2. Pour the egg mixture evenly into the molds up to the "Max" fill line.
3. Fill the egg bite maker with water according to the manufacturer's directions.
4. Place the mold in the egg bite maker and securely close the lid. Plug in the egg cooker.
5. After approximately 7 minutes, or when the green light turns off, carefully remove the egg tray from the cooker.
6. Allow the egg bites to stand for a few minutes to cool slightly.
7. Gently invert the egg bites onto a serving plate.

Tips:

- Cover and refrigerate leftover spinach and water chestnuts for up to 5 days.
- Reseal the leftover Knorr® Vegetable recipe mix and store up to the expiration date on the packet.
- If you are planning to make a spinach dip, set aside a small amount of the ingredients - enough to make these egg bites.
- A fresh small green onion, white and light green parts only can be sliced and substituted for the green onion flakes.

Avocado and Tomato Egg Bites

Creamy avocadoes, egg whites and olive oil are the magic accompaniments to fresh basil and tomatoes in these rich gems.

Serving Size: 2 egg bites | Preparation Time: 5 minutes | Cooking Time: 7 minutes

---

Ingredients:

3 tbsp.	egg whites
2 tbsp.	avocado
1 tbsp.	chopped red onions
1 tbsp.	virgin olive oil
1 tbsp.	chopped fresh basil
1 tsp.	coarse Kosher salt or sea salt
2 tbsp.	chopped tomatoes

Instructions:

1. Using a personal blender, combine the egg whites, avocado, red onions, olive oil, fresh basil, coarse salt and half of the tomatoes.
2. Sprinkle the remaining chopped tomatoes evenly divided into the egg molds.
3. Pour the egg mixture evenly into the molds up to the "Max" fill line.
4. Fill the egg bite maker with water according to the manufacturer's directions.
5. Place the mold in the egg bite maker and securely close the lid. Plug in the egg cooker.
6. After approximately 7 minutes, or when the green light turns off, carefully remove the egg tray from the cooker.
7. Allow the egg bites to stand for a few minutes to cool slightly.
8. Gently invert the egg bites onto a serving plate.

Tips:

- Serve bites on toasted slices of baguettes.
- Substitute 1 large egg for the 3 tbsp. egg whites.
- Sprinkle with more coarse salt before serving.

Mushroom & Onion Bites

Experience the magic of earthy mushrooms and sweet caramelized onions combined with a creamy havarti for savory perfection.

Serving Size: 2 egg bites | Preparation Time: 3 minutes | Cooking Time: 12 minutes

---

Ingredients:

1 tbsp.	butter
3 oz	mushrooms, about 1/2 of a small carton
1/4	onion, sliced
1	large egg
1 tbsp.	Havarti cheese
Pinch	Kosher salt and freshly ground black pepper

Instructions:

1. In a small skillet over medium heat, melt the butter. Add the mushrooms and onions. Cook stirring until the mushrooms and onions are golden brown.
2. Using a personal blender, add the mushroom and onion mixture, the egg, Havarti cheese, salt and pepper. Pulse the blender until just combined.
3. Pour the mixture evenly into the egg bite molds, filling them up to the "Max" fill line.
4. Fill the egg bite maker with water according to the manufacturer's directions.
5. Place the mold in the egg bite maker and securely close the lid. Plug in the egg cooker.
6. After approximately 7 minutes, or when the green light turns off, carefully remove the egg tray from the cooker.
7. Allow the egg bites to stand for a few minutes to cool slightly.
8. Gently invert the egg bites onto a serving plate.

Tip:

- Save a step for another dish or another batch of egg bites. Sauté a whole carton of mushrooms and a whole sliced onion until caramelized. Cover the excess mushrooms and onions. Refrigerate up to 5 days.

RED PEPPER & GOAT CHEESE MEDLEY

A delightful blend of red pepper and goat cheese combine to make the continental flavors of the unique bites.

Serving Size: 2 egg bites | Preparation Time: 3 minutes | Cooking Time: 7 minutes

---

Ingredients:

4 tbsp.	liquid egg whites
2 tbsp.	roasted red peppers, chopped
2 tbsp.	crumbled goat cheese
2 tbsp.	cream cheese, softened
Pinch	kosher salt and freshly ground black pepper

Instructions:

1. Using a personal blender, combine the egg whites, peppers, goat cheese, cream cheese, salt and pepper.
2. Pour the egg mixture evenly into the molds up to the "Max" fill line.
3. Fill the egg bite maker with water according to the manufacturer's directions.
4. Place the mold in the egg bite maker and securely close the lid. Plug in the egg cooker.
5. After approximately 7 minutes, or when the green light turns off, carefully remove the egg tray from the cooker.
6. Allow the egg bites to stand for a few minutes to cool slightly.
7. Gently invert the egg bites onto a serving plate.

Tip:

- Use a cream cheese with chives spread in place of plain cream cheese for added flavor.

Garden Fresh Zucchini & Parmesan

When the abundance of zucchini arrives in the garden and farmer's market in late summer, why not add it to your egg bites for a garden fresh treat.

Serving Size: 2 egg bites | Preparation Time: 3 minutes | Cooking Time: 7 minutes

Ingredients:

1	large egg
3 tbsp.	cottage cheese
2 tbsp.	grated zucchini
2 tbsp.	fresh grated Parmesan cheese
Pinch	Kosher salt and freshly ground black pepper

Instructions:

1. Using a personal blender, combine the egg, cottage cheese, zucchini, Parmesan, salt and pepper.
2. Pour the egg mixture evenly into the molds up to the "Max" fill line.
3. Fill the egg bite maker with water according to the manufacturer's directions.
4. Place the mold in the egg bite maker and securely close the lid. Plug in the egg cooker.
5. After approximately 7 minutes, or when the green light turns off, carefully remove the egg tray from the cooker.
6. Allow the egg bites to stand for a few minutes to cool slightly.
7. Gently invert the egg bites onto a serving plate.

Tip:

- Squeeze excess liquid out of the zucchini before adding to the blender. This will prevent your egg bites from being runny.

Mediterranean Veggie Delight

These veggie-packed egg bites feature the vibrant tastes of bell peppers, black olives, feta cheese with a whisper of almond.

Serving Size: 2 egg bites | Preparation Time: 3 minutes | Cooking Time: 7 minutes

Ingredients:

1	large egg
2 tbsp.	chopped bell peppers (assorted colors)
2 tbsp.	sliced black olives
2 tbsp.	crumbled feta cheese
1 tbsp.	almond milk
Pinch	Kosher salt and freshly ground black pepper

Instructions:

1. Using a personal blender, combine the egg, bell peppers, sliced black olives, crumbled feta cheese, almond milk, salt and pepper.
2. Pour the mixture evenly into the egg bite molds, filling them up to the "Max" fill line.
3. Fill the egg bite maker with water according to the manufacturer's directions.
4. Place the mold in the egg bite maker and securely close the lid. Plug in the egg cooker.
5. After approximately 7 minutes, or when the green light turns off, carefully remove the egg tray from the cooker.
6. Allow the egg bites to stand for a few minutes to cool slightly.
7. Gently invert the egg bites onto a serving plate.

Tip:

- Substitute 3 tbsp. liquid egg whites for the large egg.
- Whole cow's milk can be substituted for the almond milk, if desired.

PEPPERY EGG BITES

For those who love peppers, kick off your morning with peppery egg bites. Make them as spicy or tame as you like. Either way they will be an eye-opener.

Serving Size: 2 egg bites | Preparation Time: 3 minutes | Cooking Time: 7 minutes

---

Ingredients:

1	large egg
3 tbsp.	Pepper Jack cheese, shredded
2 tbsp.	chopped mini peppers (any color)
1 tbsp.	cottage cheese
1 tbsp.	dried onion flakes
Pinch	kosher salt and freshly ground black pepper
Pinch	crushed red pepper

Instructions:

1. Using a personal blender, combine the egg, pepper Jack cheese, peppers, cottage cheese, onion flakes, salt and pepper.
2. Sprinkle a bit of crushed red pepper into the bottom of the egg molds.
3. Pour the egg mixture evenly into the molds up to the "Max" fill line.
4. Fill the egg bite maker with water according to the manufacturer's directions.
5. Place the mold in the egg bite maker and securely close the lid. Plug in the egg cooker.
6. After approximately 7 minutes, or when the green light turns off, carefully remove the egg tray from the cooker.
7. Allow the egg bites to stand for a few minutes to cool slightly.
8. Gently invert the egg bites onto a serving plate.

Tips:

- In place of mini peppers, you can use chopped bell peppers.
- If you really like spicy foods, try diced jalapeños or Anaheim peppers in place of the mini peppers.

Quinoa Egg Bite Breakfast

Quinoa Egg muffins are a vegetarian and gluten-free on-the-go breakfast for a morning protein boost. They also make a power-up mid-day snack.

Serving Size: 2 egg bites | Preparation Time: 3 minutes | Cooking Time: 7 minutes

---

Ingredients:

1	large egg
2 tbsp.	cooked quinoa
2 tbsp.	shredded mozzarella
2 tbsp.	chopped fresh spinach
1 tbsp.	milk
1/8 tsp.	minced garlic
Pinch	kosher salt and freshly ground black pepper

Instructions:

1. Using a personal, combine the egg, quinoa, mozzarella, spinach, milk, garlic, salt and pepper.
2. Pour the mixture evenly into the egg bite molds up to the "Max" fill line.
3. Fill the egg bite maker with water according to the manufacturer's directions.
4. Place the mold in the cooker and close the lid. Plug in the egg cooker.
5. After about 7 minutes, or when the green light turns off, carefully remove the egg tray from the cooker.
6. Let stand a few minutes. Then invert the egg bites on to a serving plate.

Tips

- Remember to set aside 2 tbsp. of cooked quinoa from your latest quinoa recipe.

Spinach & Feta Delight

Enjoy a nutritious and flavorful breakfast with this wholesome combination of spinach and tangy feta in just 10 minutes. Get a dose of protein, vitamins and minerals at the start of your day.

Serving Size: 2 egg bites | Preparation Time: 3 minutes | Cooking Time: 7 minutes

---

Ingredients:

1	large egg
3 tbsp.	crumbled feta cheese
2 tbsp.	Greek yogurt
2 tbsp.	chopped frozen spinach, thawed
1/8 tsp.	garlic powder
Pinch	Kosher salt and freshly ground black pepper

Instructions:

1. Using a personal blender, combine the egg, feta, yogurt, spinach, garlic power, salt and pepper.
2. Pour the mixture evenly into the egg bite molds up to the "Max" fill line.
3. Fill the egg bite maker with water according to the manufacturer's directions.
4. Place the mold in the cooker and close the lid. Plug in the egg cooker.
5. After about 7 minutes, or when the green light turns off, carefully remove the egg tray from the cooker.
6. Let stand a few minutes. Then invert the egg bites on to a serving plate.

Tip:

- Squeeze excess water from the chopped spinach to avoid a watery texture.

Caprese Egg Bites

Whoever said the combination of ripe tomatoes, fresh mozzarella and fresh basil was reserved only for salads has never tried this brilliant combination for eggs. Caprese on the go? Yes please.

Serving Size: 2 egg bites | Preparation Time: 5 minutes | Cooking Time: 7 minutes

Ingredients:

3 tbsp.	liquid egg whites
2 tbsp.	whole milk
2 tbsp.	fresh mozzarella pearls
2 tbsp.	quartered cherry tomatoes
1 tbsp.	torn fresh basil leaves
Pinch	kosher salt and freshly ground black pepper
	Balsamic glaze, for drizzling

Instructions:

1. Using a personal blender, combine the egg whites, milk, mozzarella, tomatoes, basil, salt and pepper.
2. Pour the mixture evenly into the egg bite molds up to the "Max" fill line.
3. Fill the egg bite maker with water according to the manufacturer's directions.
4. Place the mold in the cooker and close the lid. Plug in the egg cooker.
5. After about 7 minutes, or when the green light turns off, carefully remove the egg tray from the cooker.
6. Let stand a few minutes. Then invert the egg bites on to a serving plate.
7. Drizzle with balsamic glaze.

Tips:

- Instead of tearing the basil leaves, cut them chiffonade style. To do this roll 3 to 4 basil leaves in a tight roll and cut them crosswise into thin slices.
- Substitute chopped sun dried tomatoes for the cherry tomatoes.

Mushroom & Swiss Sensation

This delightful blend of earthy mushrooms and creamy Swiss cheese is a savory vegetarian delight for your breakfast. Eat them warm out of the egg cooker, or pack for later. Either way, you won't be disappointed.

Serving Size: 2 egg bites | Preparation Time: 3 minutes | Cooking Time: 7 minutes

---

Ingredients:

1	large egg
1 tbsp.	unsalted butter, softened
Pinch	Kosher salt and freshly ground black pepper
3 tbsp.	shredded Swiss cheese
3	button mushrooms, chopped

Instructions:

1. Using a personal blender, combine the egg, butter, salt, pepper, 2 tbsp. Swiss cheese, and about 4 tsp. of the chopped mushrooms.
2. Sprinkle the remaining cheese and mushrooms, evenly divided, into the bottom of the egg bite molds.
3. Pour the egg mixture evenly into the egg bite molds, filling them up to the "Max" fill line.
4. Fill the egg bite maker with water according to the manufacturer's directions.
5. Place the mold in the cooker and close the lid. Plug in the egg cooker.
6. After about 7 minutes, or when the green light turns off, carefully remove the egg tray from the cooker.
7. Let stand a few minutes. Then invert the egg bites on to a serving plate.

Tips:

- 3 button mushrooms will equal about 2 tbsp. of chopped mushrooms.
- In place of fresh mushrooms, add 1 tbsp of mushroom powder. If using powder, add 1 tbsp. of heavy cream to the mix.

BROCCOLI & CHEDDAR HEAVEN

Discover the delightful pairing of broccoli and cheddar in these easy vegetarian egg bites. They are great for breakfast or a midday pick me up.

Serving Size: 2 egg bites | Preparation Time: 3 minutes | Cooking Time: 7 minutes

Ingredients:

1	large egg
1 tbsp.	cream cheese, softened
1/8 tsp.	garlic powder
Pinch	Kosher salt and freshly ground black pepper
3 tbsp.	shredded cheddar cheese
3 tbsp.	steamed chopped broccoli

Instructions:

1. Using a personal blender, combine the egg, cream cheese, garlic powder, salt and pepper. Add the shredded cheddar and the chopped broccoli; pulse the blender a couple of times until just combined.
2. Pour the egg mixture evenly into the molds up to the "Max" fill line.
3. Fill the egg bite maker with water according to the manufacturer's directions.
4. Place the mold in the cooker and close the lid. Plug in the egg cooker.
5. After about 7 minutes, or when the green light turns off, carefully remove the egg tray from the cooker.
6. Let stand a few minutes. Then invert the egg bites on to a serving plate.

Tips:

- Defrost a package of frozen chopped broccoli. Then, measure and fill ice cube trays with the broccoli to use later. Freeze or refrigerate for perfectly sized portions.
- Alternatively, set aside leftover steamed broccoli from your latest side dish.

Pesto & Sun-Dried Tomato Delight

Switch up your egg bites with this Italian inspired combination of mozzarella, sun dried tomatoes and pesto for a colorful and festive egg bite combo. They are also a festive treat to serve as an appetizer.

Serving Size: 2 egg bites | Preparation Time: 3 minutes | Cooking Time: 7 minutes

Ingredients:

1	large egg
2 tbsp.	cottage cheese
2 tsp.	pesto sauce
Pinch	Kosher salt and freshly ground black pepper
2 tbsp.	shredded mozzarella cheese
2 tbsp.	chopped sun-dried tomatoes
	Balsamic glaze (optional)

Instructions:

1. Using a personal blender, combine the egg, cottage cheese, pesto, salt and pepper. Add half of the shredded mozzarella and half of the sun-dried tomatoes; pulse the blender a couple of times until just combined.
2. Sprinkle the remaining mozzarella and sun-dried tomatoes, evenly divided, into the bottom of the egg bite molds.
3. Pour the egg mixture evenly into the molds up to the "Max" fill line.
4. Fill the egg bite maker with water according to the manufacturer's directions.
5. Place the mold in the cooker and close the lid. Plug in the egg cooker.
6. After about 7 minutes, or when the green light turns off, carefully remove the egg tray from the cooker.
7. Let stand a few minutes. Then invert the egg bites on to a serving plate.
8. Drizzle egg bites with balsamic glaze, if using.

Tip:

- Replace the large egg with 3 tbsp. of liquid egg whites if desired.

SIMPLE CHIVE &COTTAGE CHEESE

Simple certainly doesn't mean simple taste, only simple and easily prepared ingredients. The pure simplicity make these egg bites creamy, delicious and memorable.

Serving Size: 2 egg bites | Preparation Time: 3 minutes | Cooking Time: 7 minutes

Ingredients:

1	large egg
3 tbsp.	cottage cheese with chive and onion
3 tbsp.	Monterey Jack cheese, shredded
Pinch	Kosher salt and freshly ground black pepper
1 tsp.	fresh chives, chopped (optional)

Instructions:

1. Using a personal blender, combine the egg, cottage cheese, Monterey Jack, salt and pepper.
2. Pour the egg mixture evenly into the molds up to the "Max" fill line.
3. Fill the egg bite maker with water according to the manufacturer's directions.
4. Place the mold in the cooker and close the lid. Plug in the egg cooker.
5. After about 7 minutes, or when the green light turns off, carefully remove the egg tray from the cooker.
6. Let stand a few minutes. Then invert the egg bites on to a serving plate.
7. Garnish with chives, if using.

Tip:

- Replace the large egg with 3 tbsp. of liquid egg whites if desired.
- If you can't find cottage cheese with chives, add 2 tsp. of chopped chives to the blender in step 1.

TOMATO SPINACH AND FETA

These Mediterranean-inspired egg bites will transport you to the beaches of the sea, if only for a little bit. But the flavors will start your day with inspiration.

Serving Size: 2 egg bites | Preparation Time: 3 minutes | Cooking Time: 7 minutes

Ingredients:

1	large egg
1 tbsp.	cream cheese, softened
2 tbsp.	chopped fresh spinach
Pinch	kosher salt and freshly ground black pepper
2 tbsp.	chopped sun-dried tomatoes
2 tbsp.	feta cheese, crumbled

Instructions:

1. Using a personal blender, combine the egg, cream cheese, spinach, salt and pepper. Add half of the sun-dried tomatoes and half of the feta; pulse the blender a couple of times until just combined.
2. Sprinkle the remaining sun-dried tomatoes and feta, evenly divided, into the bottom of the egg bite molds.
3. Pour the egg mixture evenly into the molds up to the "Max" fill line.
4. Fill the egg bite maker with water according to the manufacturer's directions.
5. Place the mold in the cooker and close the lid. Plug in the egg cooker.
6. After about 7 minutes, or when the green light turns off, carefully remove the egg tray from the cooker.
7. Let stand a few minutes. Then invert the egg bites on to a serving plate.

Tip:

- Replace the large egg with 3 tbsp. of liquid egg whites if desired.
- For a stronger cheese infusion, use 2 tbsp. crumble bleu cheese in place of the feta.

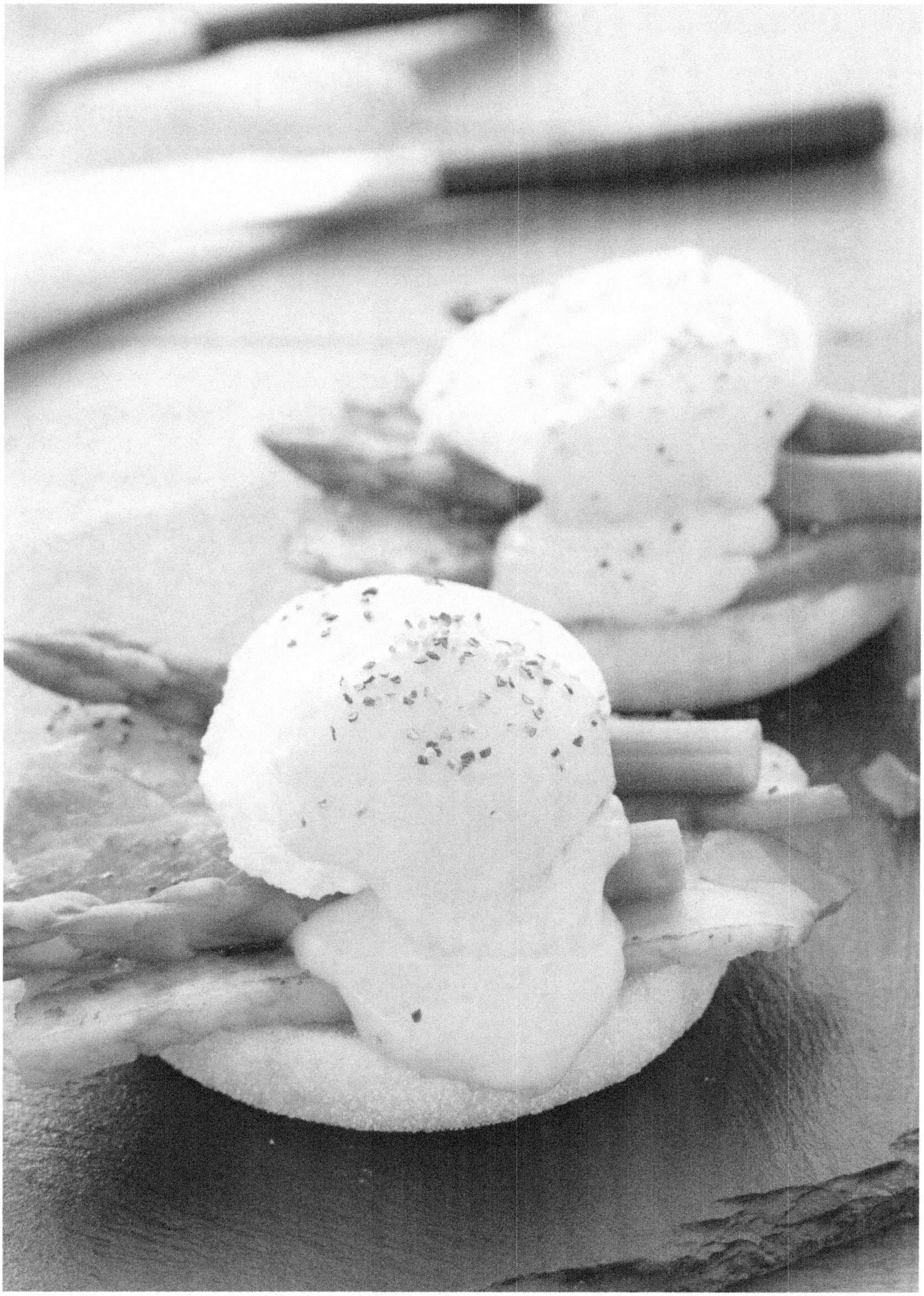

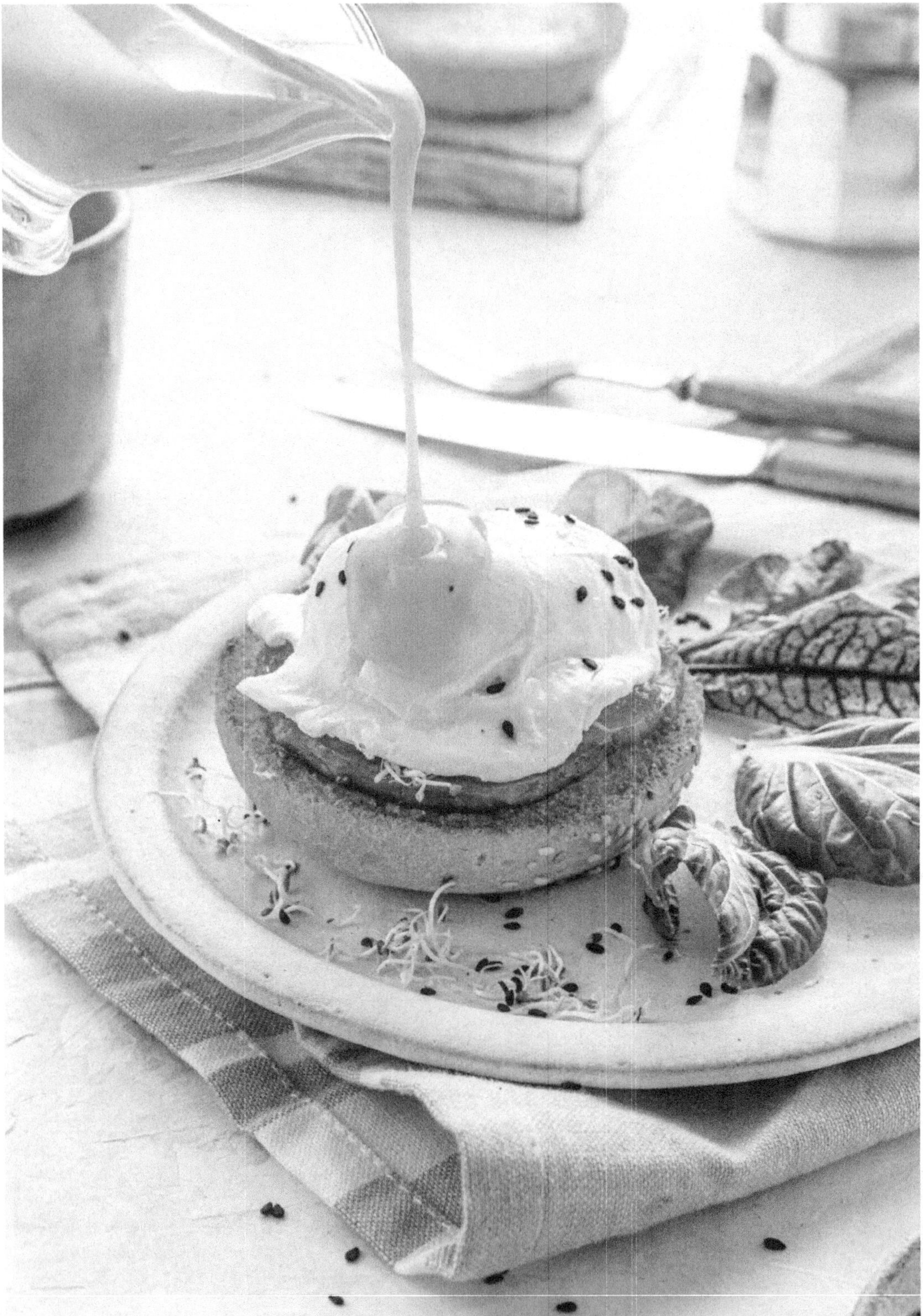

Beyond Egg Bites

When a recipe calls for a full fat dairy product such as milk, cream or cottage cheese, reducing the fat percentage can result in dryer and stiffer eggs.

BASIC POACHED EGGS

Poached eggs can be challenging to make the traditional way. But, with the Egg Bite Maker making poached eggs is simple. This is the base recipe for making poached eggs with a chart that shows how much water to add for your desired doneness.

Serving Size: 2 eggs benedict | Preparation Time: 3 minutes | Cooking Time: 7 minutes

---

Ingredients:

2 large eggs

Instructions:

1. Crack the eggs into each egg bite mold.
2. Pour water into the center well of the egg bite maker for your desired doneness. See chart below.
3. Place the mold in the cooker and close the lid. Plug in the egg cooker.
4. When the green light turns off, carefully remove the egg tray from the cooker.
5. Let eggs rest 2 minutes. Then invert egg molds onto serving plate to release eggs.

- These specific measurements apply to the Hamilton Beach egg bites maker. Follow your manufacturer's instructions for your machine.

<u>Poached Egg Doneness Guide</u>

Desired Doneness	Amount of Water
Soft	70 mL
Medium	80 mL
Hard	100 mL

Cheesecake Bites

These delightful little cheesecake bites are the perfect sized dessert. They are so simple to make in the egg bites maker too, which is a great reason for making them again and again.

Serving Size: 2 bites | Preparation Time: 3 minutes | Cooking Time: 7 minutes

Ingredients:

Filling:

4 oz	cream cheese, softened
2 tbsp.	cottage cheese
1 tbsp.	granulated sugar
1	large egg, at room temperature
1/2 tsp.	vanilla extract

Crust:

3/4 cup	graham cracker crumbs
1 tbsp.	unsalted butter, melted

Instructions:

Filling:

1. Lightly spray the egg bite molds with non-stick cooking spray.
2. Using a personal blender combine the cream cheese, cottage cheese, sugar, egg, and vanilla.
3. Pour the mixture evenly into the egg bite molds up to the "Max" fill line.

Crust:

4. In a small bowl, combine the graham cracker crumbs with the melted butter. Pat the mixture on top of the cream cheese mixture.
5. Fill the egg bite maker with water according to the manufacturer's directions.
6. Place the mold in the cooker and close the lid. Plug in the egg cooker.
7. After about 7 minutes, or when the green light turns off, carefully remove the egg tray from the cooker.
8. Let stand a few minutes. Then invert the egg bites on to a serving plate.

Tips

- You can omit the graham cracker crust if you prefer.
- Instead of the graham cracker crumbs, use crushed vanilla or chocolate wafers, shortbread cookies or gingersnaps. Alternatively, put a cooking wafer on the top without crumbling.

Quick Classic Flan

For a rich and creamy treat, this caramel custard known as flan, is the most enjoyable quick and easy dessert.

Serving Size: 2 flans | Preparation Time: 3 minutes | Cooking Time: 7 minutes

Ingredients:

2 tbsp.	caramel syrup
1/4 cup	whole milk
1	large egg yolk, at room temperature
½ tbsp.	granulated sugar
2 drops	vanilla extract
	Fresh raspberries, for garnish, optional

Instructions:

1. Lightly spray the egg bite molds with non-stick cooking spray.
2. Spoon 1 tbsp. of caramel syrup into the bottom of each egg bite mold.
3. In a small saucepan over medium heat, add the milk and heat until steaming.
4. Meanwhile, in a small bowl whisk the egg yolk, sugar and vanilla together. Continue whisking and slowly pour in a little hot milk. While still whisking, slowly pour in the remaining milk.
5. Spoon the custard mixture into each mold up to the "Max" fill line.
6. Pour 100 ml of water into the center well of the egg bite maker.
7. Place the mold in the cooker and close the lid. Plug in the egg cooker.
8. After about 7 minutes, or when the green light turns off, carefully remove the egg tray from the cooker.
9. Let stand a few minutes. Then invert the flan on to a serving plate. Garnish with raspberries, if using.

Tip:

- Substitute an equal amount of blackberries or chopped fresh strawberries for the raspberries.

Key Lime Pie

Originating in the Florida Keys, this famous pie has seen many iterations, but its true heart — a combination of Key limes and a sweet cream custard — remains the same. Serve it dolloped with whipped cream, if desired.

Serving Size: 2 egg bites | Preparation Time: 3 minutes | Cooking Time: 7 minutes

---

Ingredients:

2	large egg yolks
5 tbsp.	sweetened condensed milk
2-½ tbsp.	fresh key lime juice

Instructions:

1. Using a personal blender or hand whisking in a bowl, blend the egg yolks until light yellow. Add the sweetened condensed milk and the key lime juice, pulsing or whisking until combined.
2. Pour the mixture evenly into the egg bite molds, filling them up to the "Max" fill line.
3. Place the mold in the egg bite maker and securely close the lid. Plug in the egg cooker.
4. After approximately 7 minutes, or when the green light turns off, carefully remove the egg tray from the cooker.
5. Allow the egg bites to stand for a few minutes to cool slightly.
6. Gently invert the egg bites onto a serving plate.

Tips

- If you are unable to find fresh Key limes, you can use bottled juice, often called Key West lime juice (not Key lime juice). It can be found with the bottles of lemon and lime juice in your grocery store.
- The leftover egg whites can be refrigerated for up to 2 days. Use them in one of the many egg white bites recipes in this book.

Eggs Benedict

Nothing says decadent breakfast better than Eggs Benedict. If you have been intimidated by poaching eggs and making hollandaise, be assured the egg bites maker makes poaching eggs super easy. Combine them with the foolproof Hollandaise sauce recipe that follows.

Serving Size: 2 eggs benedict | Preparation Time: 3 minutes | Cooking Time: 7 minutes

Ingredients:

2	large eggs
1	English muffin
2	slices of Canadian bacon
2/3 cup	hollandaise sauce (recipe on the following page)

Instructions:

1. Crack the eggs into each egg bite mold.
2. Pour 70 ml of water into the center well of the egg bite maker for soft poached eggs. (see tip)
3. Place the mold in the cooker and close the lid. Plug in the egg cooker.
4. When the green light turns off, carefully remove the egg tray from the cooker.
5. Meanwhile, toast 2 halves of an English muffin.
6. In a small skillet, heat the Canadian bacon.
7. Place the toasted muffins on serving plates. Top each with a slice of Canadian bacon and a poached egg.
8. Spoon the hollandaise sauce on top of each poached egg. Serve warm.

Tip

- Follow the egg doneness chart at the beginning of this chapter for soft, medium or hard poached eggs.

Easy Hollandaise Sauce

Enjoy this quick and easy golden yellow hollandaise sauce drizzled over eggs Benedict, asparagus, roasted potatoes, or baked salmon. This easy foolproof sauce recipe is ideal for home cooks.

Serving Size: 2/3 cup sauce | Preparation Time: 3 minutes | Cooking Time: 3 minutes

---

Ingredients:

2	egg yolks
1 tsp.	water
1 tsp.	lemon juice from 1 lemon
	Kosher salt
8 tbsp.	unsalted butter (1 stick)
Pinch	cayenne pepper (optional)

This recipe was inspired by inspired by J. Kenji López-Alt.

Instructions:

1. In a cup just wide enough to fit the head of an immersion blender, combine egg yolks, water, lemon juice, and a pinch of salt.
2. In a small saucepan with a spout, melt butter over high heat, swirling constantly, until foaming subsides.
3. Place head of immersion blender into the bottom of the cup and turn it on. With the blender continuously running, slowly pour hot butter into the blended eggs in a steady stream of little droplets to emulsify the mixture.
4. Continue pouring until all butter is added. The sauce should be creamy and thick enough to coat a spoon but still flow off of it. If it is too thick, whisk in a small amount of warm water, 1 tbsp. at a time, to thin it out to the desired consistency.
5. Season to taste with salt and a pinch of cayenne pepper, if using.
6. Spoon the warm sauce immediately over the poached eggs.

Tips

- You can make the sauce up to 1 hour in advance and keep it warm by placing the cup in a bowl of warm (not hot) water.
- Hollandaise sauce cannot be refrigerated and reheated later.

Cheesy Ramen With Poached Eggs

This Cheesy Ramen Noodles recipe combines the comforting familiarity of a package of ramen noodles with the rich creaminess of a perfectly poached egg and a delightful layer of melted cheese. It is classic Korean comfort food that is pure cheesy goodness.

Serving Size: 1 | Preparation Time: 1 minute | Cooking Time: 6 minutes

---

Ingredients:

1	large egg
1 pkg.	ramen noodles, chicken flavor
1/2 tsp.	butter, softened
2 slices	American cheese, room temperature
1	green onion light green middle part only, thinly sliced diagonally
1/4 tsp.	toasted sesame seeds
	Chili garlic sauce (optional)

Instructions:

1. Crack the egg into an egg bite mold.
2. Pour 70 ml of water into the center well of the egg bite maker for soft poached eggs. (See the Poached Egg Doneness chart for other options.)
3. Place the mold in the cooker and close the lid. Plug in the egg cooker.
4. When the green light turns off, carefully remove the egg tray from the cooker.
5. Meanwhile, in a medium saucepan over medium-high heat, add 2-½ cups water and heat until boiling. Add the ramen noodles and cook for 2 minutes. Add the flavor packet, stir, and continue cooking for another 30 seconds or until noodles are softened.
6. Carefully transfer the ramen and broth to a serving bowl. Stir in the butter. Add the cheese and poached egg to the top. Garnish with green onions. Sprinkle with toasted sesame seeds, if using.
7. Serve hot with chili garlic sauce on the side, if using.

Tip:

- Use any flavor of Ramen noodles you prefer.

Smoked Salmon Benedict

Rich, smoky salmon is layered on English muffins and topped with a delicately poached egg. All topped with creamy hollandaise sauce. Serve with a side of fresh berries and you have a very special brunch.

Serving Size: 4 | Preparation Time: 3 minutes | Cooking Time: 7 minutes

Ingredients:

2	English muffins
2 tbsp.	butter
4	slices smoked salmon (about 4 oz.)
4	large eggs
1 tbsp.	capers
	Freshly ground black pepper
Hollandaise	
2	egg yolks
1 tsp.	water
1 tsp.	lemon juice from 1 lemon
	Kosher salt
8 tbsp.	unsalted butter (1 stick)
1 tsp.	Dijon mustard

Instructions:

1. Toast the halves of the English muffins. Butter the toasted halves and place them on serving plates.
2. Lay the slices of salmon, evenly divided, among the toasted muffins.
3. Crack 2 of the eggs into the egg bite mold.
4. Pour 70 ml of water into the center well of the egg bite maker for soft poached eggs. (see Tip)
5. Place the mold in the cooker and close the lid. Plug in the egg cooker.
6. When the green light turns off, carefully remove the egg tray from the cooker. Let eggs rest for 2 minutes. Then place them on top of the salmon.
7. Repeat steps 3 to 6 with the remaining eggs.

Hollandaise Sauce:

8. Meanwhile, in a cup just wide enough to fit the head of an immersion blender, combine egg yolks, water, lemon juice, and a pinch of salt.
9. In a small saucepan with a spout, melt butter over high heat, swirling constantly, until foaming subsides.
10. Place the head of the immersion blender into the bottom of the cup and turn it on. With the blender continuously running, slowly pour hot butter into the blended eggs in a steady stream of little droplets to emulsify the mixture.

...Continued next page

Smoked Salmon Benedict (continued)

Instructions (continued):

11. Continue pouring until all butter is added. The sauce should be creamy and thick enough to coat a spoon but still flow off it. If it is too thick, whisk in a small amount of warm water, 1 tbsp. at a time, to thin it out to the desired consistency.
12. Season to taste with salt and a pinch of cayenne pepper, if using.
13. Spoon the warm sauce immediately over the poached eggs.
14. Garnish with capers and a twist of black pepper.

Tips

- Follow the egg doneness chart for soft, medium or hard poached eggs. These specific measurements apply to the Hamilton Beach egg bites maker. Follow your manufacturer's instructions for your machine.

Gluten-Free Eggs Florentine

An amazing combination of spinach, beefsteak tomatoes and poached eggs, blanketed in a cheesy spinach blend. No muffin needed.

Serving Size: 4 | Preparation Time: 3 minutes | Cooking Time: 12 minutes

Ingredients:

4	slices prosciutto, coarsely chopped
3 tbsp.	olive oil
1	small onion, finely chopped
3 cloves	garlic, minced
5 cups	baby spinach
1/4 tsp.	ground nutmeg
2/3 cup	grated Pecorino Romano
	Kosher salt
	Black pepper
2	beefsteak tomatoes, sliced 1-inch-thick
4	large eggs

Substitution:

You can use 1/2 cup frozen spinach in place of the fresh spinach. Defrost the spinach and squeeze the spinach to get rid of excess moisture.

Instructions:

1. In a medium skillet over medium-high heat, add the prosciutto and cook, stirring, until crispy. Remove from the skillet. Set aside and let cool.
2. In the same skillet add the oil and heat until shimmering. Add the onion and cook, stirring, 5 minutes or until soft. Add the garlic and cook, stirring, 30 seconds or until fragrant. Add the spinach and nutmeg and cook until the spinach has wilted, about 1 to 2 minutes. Remove the pan from the heat and stir in the cheese.
3. Place the tomato slices onto serving plates and season with salt and pepper.
4. Spoon 1/4 of the wilted spinach mixture over each tomato slice.
5. Meanwhile, crack 2 of the eggs into the egg bite mold.
6. Pour 70 ml of water into the center well of the egg bite maker for soft poached eggs. (see Tip)
7. Place the mold in the cooker and close the lid. Plug in the egg cooker.
8. When the green light turns off, remove the egg tray from the cooker. Let eggs rest for 2 minutes. Then, place them on top of the creamed spinach and tomatoes.
9. Repeat steps 4 to 7 with the remaining eggs.
10. Crumble the cooked prosciutto and sprinkle over the eggs.

New Orleans Style Eggs Sardou

Folk lore tells us that Eggs Benedict was originally created in New York as a hangover cure. So, no one should be surprised that a variation of this famous recipe began in the French Quarter.

Serving Size: 2 | Preparation Time: 3 minutes | Cooking Time: 30 minutes

---

Ingredients:

5 tsp.	butter, divided
1 tbsp.	minced shallots
1/2 tsp.	minced garlic
1 tbsp.	all-purpose flour
3/4 cup	whole milk
5 oz	fresh baby spinach leaves (about 2-1/2 cups)
	Kosher salt and freshly ground black pepper
4	whole canned artichoke bottoms (from one 14-ounce can)
4	eggs
1/8 tsp.	hot sauce
Hollandaise	
2	egg yolks
1 tsp.	water
1 tsp.	lemon juice
	Kosher salt and freshly ground black pepper
8 tbsp.	unsalted butter (1 stick)

Instructions:

1. In a small saucepan over medium heat, melt 3 tsp. of butter. Add shallots and cook, stirring, 3 minutes or until softened. Add the garlic and cook, stirring, 30 seconds. Slowly whisk in the flour and cook until lightly browned. Slowly add the milk, whisking continuously, until no lumps remain. Bring to a simmer and cook, stirring often, 5 minutes or until thickened.
2. Add the spinach and stir until wilted. Simmer over low heat, stirring occasionally, 15 minutes or until thickened and creamy. Stir in hot sauce. Season with salt and pepper.
3. Meanwhile, melt the remaining 2 tsp. butter in a small skillet over medium heat. Add artichoke bottoms and cook, stirring, until heated but not browned, about 5 minutes.
4. Meanwhile, poach according to the Basic Poached Eggs recipe at the beginning of this chapter. Soft poached is ideal for this recipe.
5. Divide creamed spinach between 2 plates, place 2 warmed artichoke bottoms on top of each portion of spinach. Add the poached eggs on top of the artichokes.

Hollandaise Sauce:

6. Meanwhile, in a cup just wide enough to fit the head of an immersion blender, combine egg yolks, water, lemon juice, and a pinch of salt.

...Continued next page

NEW ORLEANS STYLE EGGS SARDOU (CONTINUED)

Instructions (continued):

7. In a small saucepan with a spout, melt butter over high heat, swirling constantly, until foaming subsides.
8. Place the head of the immersion blender into the bottom of the cup and turn it on. With the blender continuously running, slowly pour hot butter into the blended eggs in a steady stream of little droplets to emulsify the mixture.
9. Continue pouring until all butter is added. The sauce should be creamy and thick enough to coat a spoon but still flow off it. If it is too thick, whisk in a small amount of warm water, 1 tbsp. at a time, to thin it out to the desired consistency.
10. Season to taste with kosher salt and black pepper.
11. Pour hollandaise sauce over the top of the eggs.
12. Serve warm with hot sauce on the side.

Tips

- Follow the egg doneness chart at the beginning of this chapter for soft, medium or hard poached eggs.

California Eggs Benedict

Eggs Benedict California style with fresh avocados, tomato, and bacon with a prepared Hollandaise sauce. Delicious and a good source of fiber and an excellent source of vitamins and minerals.

Serving Size: 2 | Preparation Time: 3 minutes | Cooking Time: 30 minutes

---

Ingredients:

1	English muffin
2 slices	Canadian bacon, warmed
1	large vine-ripened tomato, into 4 thick slices
1	ripe, avocado peeled, seeded and sliced
2	large eggs
Hollandaise	
2	egg yolks
1 tsp.	water
1 tsp.	lemon juice
	Kosher salt and freshly ground black pepper
8 tbsp.	unsalted butter (1 stick)

Instructions:

1. Toast muffin halves. Place each half on a serving plate.
2. Top each with 1 slice warm Canadian bacon, 2 slices tomato, and 1/2 of the avocado slices.
3. Meanwhile, poach eggs according to the Basic Poached Eggs recipe using 70 ml water.
4. Top each California Benedict with a poached egg.

Hollandaise Sauce:

5. Meanwhile, in a cup just wide enough to fit the head of an immersion blender, combine egg yolks, water, lemon juice, and a pinch of salt.
6. In a small saucepan with a spout, melt butter over high heat, swirling constantly, until foaming subsides.
7. Place the head of the immersion blender into the bottom of the cup and turn it on. With the blender continuously running, slowly pour hot butter into the blended eggs in a steady stream of little droplets to emulsify the mixture.
8. Continue pouring until all butter is added. The sauce should be creamy and thick enough to coat a spoon but still flow off it. If it is too thick, whisk in a small amount of warm water, 1 tbsp. at a time, to thin it out to the desired consistency.

...Continued next page

CALIFORNIA EGGS BENEDICT (CONTINUED)

Instructions (continued):

9. Season to taste with kosher salt and black pepper.
10. Spoon warm Hollandaise sauce over each serving.
11. Serve warm.

Tips

- Serve with fresh fruit.
- Follow the egg doneness chart at the beginning of this chapter for soft, medium or hard poached eggs.

Crab Cake Eggs Benedict

A twist on the classic Eggs Benedict is a dish called Eggs Royale which substitutes crab meat for the Canadian bacon. Here we replace the English muffin and crab meat with a crab cake.

Serving Size: 2 eggs benedict | Preparation Time: 3 minutes | Cooking Time: 7 minutes

---

Ingredients:

2	prepared crab cakes
2	large eggs
2/3 cup	hollandaise sauce (recipe on the following page)
Hollandaise	
2	egg yolks
1 tsp.	water
1 tsp.	lemon juice
	Kosher salt and freshly ground black pepper
8 tbsp.	unsalted butter (1 stick)

Instructions:

1. Prepare the crab cakes according to the package directions.
2. Crack the eggs into each egg bite mold.
3. Pour 70 ml of water into the center well of the egg bite maker for soft poached eggs.
4. Place the mold in the cooker and close the lid. Plug in the egg cooker.
5. When the green light turns off, carefully remove the egg tray from the cooker. Let stand 3 minutes.
6. Place poached eggs on top of each crab cake.

Hollandaise Sauce:

7. Meanwhile, in a cup just wide enough to fit the head of an immersion blender, combine egg yolks, water, lemon juice, and a pinch of salt.
8. In a small saucepan with a spout, melt butter over high heat, swirling constantly, until foaming subsides.
9. Place the head of the immersion blender into the bottom of the cup and turn it on. With the blender continuously running, slowly pour hot butter into the blended eggs in a steady stream of little droplets to emulsify the mixture.

...Continued next page

CRAB CAKE EGGS BENEDICT (CONTINUED)

Instructions (continued):

10. Continue pouring until all butter is added. The sauce should be creamy and thick enough to coat a spoon but still flow off it. If it is too thick, whisk in a small amount of warm water, 1 tbsp. at a time, to thin it out to the desired consistency.
11. Season to taste with kosher salt and black pepper.
12. Spoon warm Hollandaise sauce over each serving.
13. Serve warm.

Tip

- Crab cakes can be found in the seafood and fish section of your grocery store or in the frozen foods section.
- You can add toasted English muffin halves under the crab. if you prefer.

SMASHED POTATOES WITH EGGS

This recipe is the final recipe in the book, not only because it takes longer to prepare than my other recipes, but because it is a brilliant example of how you can make a delightful brunch or dinner with a simple poached egg.

Serving Size: 2 | Preparation Time: 3 minutes | Cooking Time: 40 minutes

---

Ingredients:

1 lb.	small red potatoes, peeled
	Kosher salt
2 sprigs	fresh rosemary, divided
3 cloves	garlic, divided
1/2	lemon. juice and grated zest of
3 tbsp.	extra-virgin olive oil
Pinch	crushed red chili flakes
	Grape seed or canola oil for frying
2	large eggs

Inspired by Florence Fabricant, from the NY Times.

Instructions:

1. Boil potatoes in salted water with 1 sprig of rosemary and 2 cloves of garlic, 15 to 20 minutes or until tender. Drain potatoes and discard rosemary and garlic.
2. Place potatoes on a cutting board. Use the the bottom of a glass bowl to lightly crush them, keeping them as intact as possible.
3. Vinaigrette: Strip leaves from remaining rosemary sprig and chop. Mince remaining garlic clove. Place in a dish with lemon juice and zest and whisk in olive oil and chili flakes. Season with salt. Set aside.
4. Preheat oven to 200 degrees F.
5. Line a small baking sheet with layers of paper towels.
6. In a 10-inch skillet over medium-high heat, add grape seed or canola oil to 1/2 -inch and heat until shimmering. Add the smashed potatoes and fry, turning once, until golden brown and crusty. Season with salt, transfer to baking sheet and place in the oven.

...Continued next page

SMASHED POTATOES WITH EGGS (CONTINUED)

Instructions (continued):

7. Meanwhile, poach eggs according to the Basic Poached Eggs recipe using 70 ml water.
8. Divide potatoes between two warm plates, whisk the vinaigrette again, and drizzle about half of it over the potatoes.
9. Add a poached egg onto each smashed potato serving.
10. Drizzle eggs with the rest of the vinaigrette and serve.

Tips

- Feel free to double the eggs.
- You can add other brunch-worthy food alongside, like smoked salmon, bacon or cured ham.
- You don't need to peel the potatoes if you prefer not to. However, there will be some loose pieces of skin that are left over. If you don't mind that, you can skip the step to peel the potatoes.
- In place of frying the potatoes in step 6, brush them lightly with the oil and cook in a 400 degree F oven for 20 minutes, turning once.

Avocado Bruschetta with Prosciutto and Poached Eggs

Serving Size: 4 | Preparation Time: 3 minutes | Cooking Time: 10 minutes

Ingredients:

4	eggs
4	thickly cut slices of ciabatta loaf
	Olive oil
1	garlic clove, halved
2	ripe avocados
8	slices prosciutto

Instructions:

1. Preheat broiler with rack in top position.
2. Poach eggs according to the Basic Poached Eggs recipe using 70 ml water. Set aside the first 2 eggs on a plate lined with kitchen paper to drain. Cover the eggs loosely with foil to keep warm and poach the remaining 2 eggs.
3. Brush ciabatta slices on both sides with the olive oil. Arrange slices on a baking sheet. Broil, turning once, 3 to 4 minutes or until toasted and golden on both sides.
4. Set aside to cool slightly, then rub each slice all over with garlic. Set on 4 serving plates.
5. Meanwhile, halve, stone and peel each avocado. Cut each avocado half into 2 wedges and layer 2 wedges on each garlic ciabatta slice, along with 2 slices of prosciutto. Top each bruschetta with a still-warm poached egg and season with salt and freshly ground black pepper to serve.

Tip:

- If you have a larger egg bites maker that cooks 4 or more bites, there is no need to set them on a lined plate in step 2. As they will all be done at the same time and ready to serve.

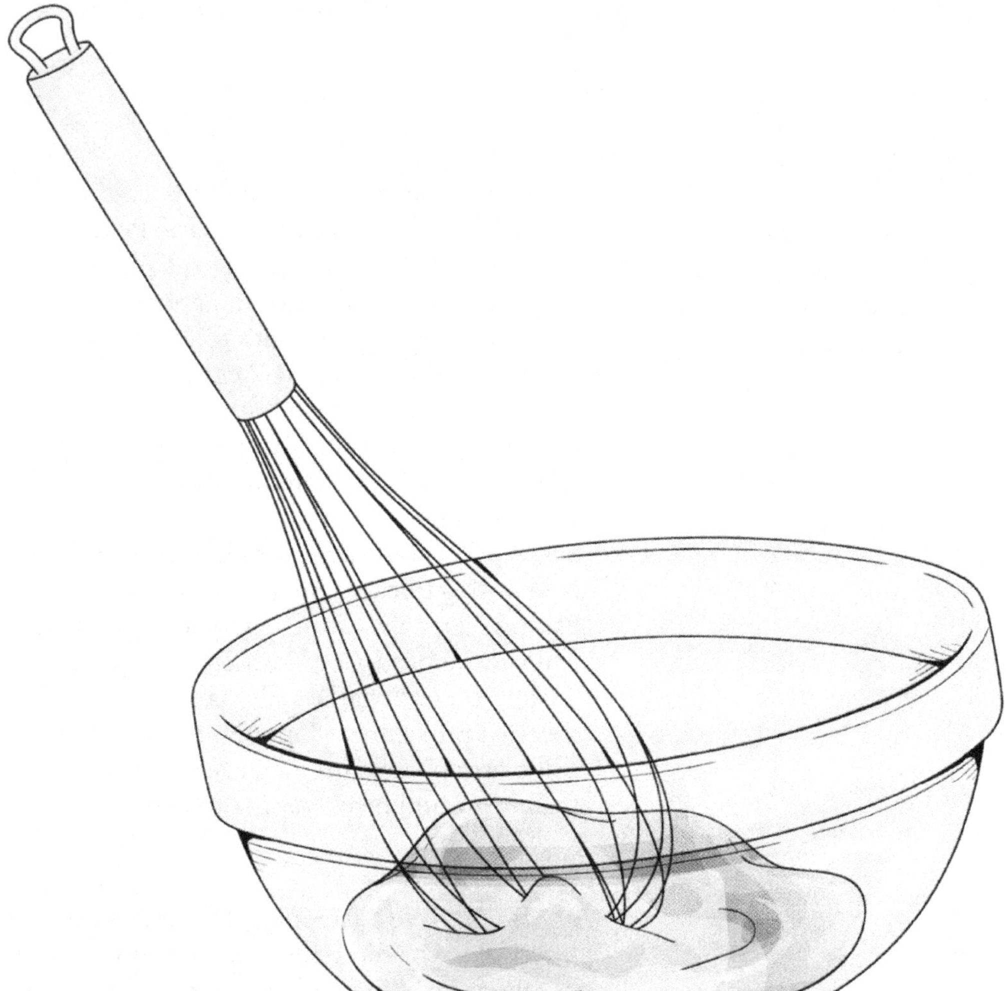

FROM THE AUTHOR

I cannot thank you enough for your interest in my Egg Bites Cookbook. I sincerely hope you have found recipes that you love and will keep as your favorites. Even more, I hope I have made making a quick and delicious breakfast much easier for you.

I would love to hear from you. If you like the recipes you've tried and would recommend these to others, please write a review on Amazon.com

If you would like to get more recipes and easy, delicious recipes, join me at MavenCookery.com

Check out more of my #1 Best Selling Cookbooks on Amazon.

I appreciate you being my customer!

Thank you, Marilyn

Marilyn

Made in United States
North Haven, CT
10 November 2026

22095607R00046